Dear

It is my pleasure to share with you my 1st book. I hope you will find it useful.

Ibrahim
Al-Zu'bi

Dubai 8/8/2020

HOW TO 'NET' POSITIVE

Ibrahim Al-Zu'bi

Copyright © 2020 Ibrahim Al-Zu'bi.

All rights reserved. No part of this book may be reproduced, stored, or transmitted by any means—whether auditory, graphic, mechanical, or electronic—without written permission of the author, except in the case of brief excerpts used in critical articles and reviews. Unauthorized reproduction of any part of this work is illegal and is punishable by law.

Because of the dynamic nature of the Internet, any web addresses or links contained in this book may have changed since publication and may no longer be valid. The views expressed in this work are solely those of the author and do not necessarily reflect the views of the publisher, and the publisher hereby disclaims any responsibility for them.

Any people depicted in stock imagery provided by Getty Images are models, and such images are being used for illustrative purposes only. Certain stock imagery © Getty Images.

ISBN: 978-1-4834-9455-5 (sc)
ISBN: 978-1-4834-9454-8 (hc)
ISBN: 978-1-4834-9453-1 (e)

Library of Congress Control Number: 2018914465

rev. date: 01/15/2020

Table of Contents

Foreword v

Chapter 1 - Business and the society: from social responsibility to shared value 1

Chapter 2 - Business and the society: quantifying the impact 33

Chapter 3 - Majid Al Futtaim: doing well by doing good 77

Chapter 4 - A blueprint for Net Positive: helping businesses give more than they take 104

Chapter 5 - Sustainability in the age of the Fourth Industrial Revolution 132

Foreword

It is my pleasure to introduce the book How To 'Net' Positive.

Today, sustainability is no longer a charity agenda, or a corporate social responsibility item to be ticked-off the list, but an engine for growth. Indeed, many businesses are thriving as a result of placing sustainability as part of their core business. As the world continues to face challenges associated with growing population, increasing resource constraints and mounting environmental issues notably climate change, only businesses that incorporate sustainability into their business operations will stand the test of time.

This is something that the UAE leaders have long known. The UAE is celebrating the "Year of Zayed" in 2018, marking the 100th anniversary of the founding father of the country, the late His Highness Sheikh Zayed bin Sultan Al Nahyan, who was a visionary on environmental sustainability. Long before the emergence of the term "sustainable development" or "green economy", Sheikh Zayed instilled in us the core value of nature conservation, to take only what is needed, and to preserve for future generations in all what we do today.

Today, these concepts are deeply embedded in our national strategies, such as the UAE Vision 2021, UAE Centennial 2071, National Climate Change Plan 2050 and Green Agenda 2030, and implemented through innovative initiatives driven by partnerships amongst the government, private sector and academia, in the pursuit of economic diversification and environmental protection, which we believe goes hand in hand.

The UAE's efforts are very much in line with the Paris Climate Agreement and the UN Sustainable Development Goals to 2030 which unite the world toward a sustainable development path. Business has a critical role in the delivery of these two major global milestones, which also provide key reference points for business engagement, for example, in the form of Nationally Determined Contributions under the Paris Agreement for investment opportunities.

Against these global and local circumstances, this book is recommended to those interested in finding out how some of the region's successful enterprises have embraced sustainability, integrated it into their business models, and achieved tangible results in doing so.

Majid Al Futtaim's Net Positive by 2040 initiative is particularly noteworthy. "Net Positive" essentially means doing more good than harm, creating positive impact on the world. Majid Al Futtaim is focusing on carbon and water, which is both highly relevant to this region which faces high temperatures in summer months and limited fresh water resources. By introducing efficiency measures, emissions reduction measures and innovative renewable energy and water generation technologies in phases, Majid Al Futtaim is expected to play a catalyst role for others to follow suit.

As the UAE Minister of Climate Change and Environment, I cannot stress strong enough how important it is for the business sector to be part of our quest for sustainable development. The case studies featured in this book are an inspiration to all those who seek to realize sustainable development.

Let us all work together hand in hand for a sustainable future for all.

H.E. Dr. Thani Ahmed Al Zeyoudi
UAE Minister of Climate Change and Environment

Chapter 1

Business and the society: from social responsibility to shared value

Nine billion humans vs. the environment

Since the dawn of time, humans have been expanding into a variety of environments to establish and grow their presence and control. This expansion has altered the ecological equilibrium of these environments on a continuous basis[1], and the history of life on earth became the history of human interaction with the environment. In the pre-industrial society, the impact of human civilization on the environment was mainly through anthropogenic fire, agriculture, and the extinction of certain types of megafauna[2]. However, the scale and extent of environmental impact spurred by the Industrial Revolution was unprecedented, and now promises to accelerate even more as we stand at the beginning of the 4th Industrial Revolution[3].

The Industrial Revolution, which started in the mid-1700s in Great Britain, marked a milestone in the history of the human-ecology interaction. It was not until 100 years after the onset of the Industrial Revolution that humans started realizing its profound impact. The replacement of wind, water and wood with fossil fuels transformed the way people lived and consumed energy. While this undoubtedly led to huge gains in production capacity and manufacturing outputs, it came at the expense of the environment. Contamination of the air, land, rivers, and the seas with dangerous materials was a natural side effect[4].

In addition, coal and other fossil fuels were incorrectly assumed to be unlimited in supply, leading to over-exploitation over the centuries[5].

Furthermore, the Industrial Revolution also spurred rapid and unparalleled growth in human population around the world. At the beginning of the first millennium AD, total human population was estimated to be between 150 and 200 million. In the year 1000, this number had increased to 300 million. In the mid-1700s, just before the advent of the Industrial Revolution the world's human population grew to 700 million - a number that was expected to reach 1 billion by 1800. The Industrial Revolution improved living standards and advanced medicine, resulting in the population boom which would carry forward into the subsequent centuries. By 1927, the world population reached 2 billion, doubling the number of humans in 100 years since the beginning of the Industrial Revolution. By the dawn of the 21st century, world population had grown exponentially to 6 billion – an extraordinary 400% increase since the 20th century. In 2017, the world population is estimated to be 7.2 billion, which is approximately 9 times the number of people at the dawn of the Industrial Revolution. The increase in population continues today, with 75 million people being added every year. Projections show that by 2020, world population will hit the 8 billion mark, increasing to 9 billion in the next twenty years or so. This will have a profound impact on our environment. This impact will undoubtedly be negative on a large scale if these 9 billion people behave and consume the way we did in the late 20th century.

In today's consumer driven capitalist world, these billions of people need an economic foothold which allows them to live a healthy and decent life. Those under the poverty line are struggling to merely survive and want greater access to food, shelter, safe water and healthcare. Those just above the poverty line are seeking ways to create better prospects for their children's future. People in high-income economies are hoping for more technological developments that will further improve their health and well-being. These varying aspirations all come together in a world that is interconnected (some even say hyperconnected) in the areas of trade, capital, technologies, human migration, social networks and production flows[6]. The forces of globalization, consumerism, and medical advances can only mean one thing: more people on earth will continue to grow in numbers, consuming more of its resources, and aspiring to raise their economic standards.

This is reflected in the scale of the world economy which stood at over US$ 107 trillion (Global World Output in 2016), roughly 200 times larger than before the Industrial Revolution began. With the advent of the 4th Industrial Revolution[7] today, the overall size of the economy is expected to grow even faster, and so will the gap in income distribution, between countries, and within countries. In 2017, while longevity and quality of life are improving in high-income countries, more than one billion people around the world live in extreme poverty (under US$ 1.25/ day), struggling for mere survival from one day to the next[8]. Nearly half of these people live in India and China, and more than 85% live in 20 countries[9].

However, global inequality of incomes is not the only challenge the world faces today as its population grows. The growth is inevitably entwined with the demand for natural and manmade resources, energy, food, and housing. This implies added pressure on the environment, which is already suffering from the adverse impacts of excessive production, over-exploitation of natural resources, and the resulting increase in dangerous by-products. According to a research conducted by World Wildlife Fund, the demand on the planet's natural resources has doubled in the last half-century, with the major part of this burden falling on poorer countries[10]. Currently, the world's economic superpowers - the USA, UK, Japan, Germany and China – consume more than double the amount of resources they produce. The World Wildlife Fund estimated that if the world continues to consume and produce at its current rate and trends are not reversed, by 2030 humankind will require resources worth two Planets Earth to sustain human activity[11]. Unfortunately, this is not an option, and something has to change!

It is now clear to most business leaders and policy makers that the world economy is creating complex environmental challenges on various overlapping fronts. Human activity is leading to climate change, limiting the availability of fresh water, altering the oceans' chemical and acidic makeup, and changing the habitats of other species co-existing with humans on the planet. Humankind now lives in what Paul Crutzen describes as the Anthropocene - an epoch where the physical environment is driven by humans themselves[12]. This concept is closely related to the "planetary boundaries" identified by a group of 9 ecologists in 2009[13]. These ecologists found that human activity was placing great stress on the global ecosystem by trespassing key environmental thresholds such as climate change, acidification of the oceans, release of nitrogen and phosphorous into the environment, rapid freshwater depletion and deforestation.

The changes in the global ecosystem are not only evident anecdotally in each environmental realm, they are quantifiable. One famous example is the global temperature which has been rising 1.7% every year since 1980. Another is the carbon dioxide levels in the air which are at their highest in 650,000 years. Arctic sea ice and glaciers are melting at an alarming rate (3.5%-4.1% every decade since 1979). Global flooding is on the rise and is expected to triple by 2030. Rising temperatures and unpredictable patterns of rainfall led to various instances of diminishing crop yields and challenges pertaining to food security and malnutrition in developing countries. Global incidences of water-transmitted, vector-borne and respiratory diseases are also on the rise as a result of climatic changes. This list goes on and on, and is fairly alarming.

Today, coupled with a steep economic growth curve, human neglect of the environment is rampant, and the results are evident in the rising number of natural catastrophes around the world[14], as well as the rise of complex challenges that have left nations looking for solutions and ways to better govern our planet and environment.

A global response to global challenges

As the 20th century was coming to an end, and to counter income inequalities and eradicate extreme poverty, the United Nations identified eight international development goals which were to be met by 2015. Launched in the year 2000, these Millennium Development Goals (MDGs), emphasized reducing the incidence of extreme poverty and hunger, promoting human development (health and education) and gender equality, and ensuring environmental sustainability. The table below outlines the main MDG focus areas and targets.

	Millennium Development Goals	
	Goals	Targets
1.	Eradicate extreme poverty and hunger	• Halve, between 1990 and 2015, the proportion of people whose income is less than $1.25 a day • Achieve full and productive employment and decent work for all, including women and young people • Halve, between 1990 and 2015, the proportion of people who suffer from hunger
2.	Achieve universal primary education	• Ensure that, by 2015, children everywhere, boys and girls alike, will be able to complete a full course of primary schooling
3.	Promote gender equality and empower women	• Eliminate gender disparity in primary and secondary education, preferably by 2005, and in all levels of education no later than 2015
4.	Reduce child mortality	• Reduce by two thirds, between 1990 and 2015, the under-five mortality rate
5.	Improve maternal health	• Reduce by three quarters, between 1990 and 2015, the maternal mortality ratio • Achieve, by 2015, universal access to reproductive health

Millennium Development Goals		
	Goals	Targets
6.	Combat HIV/AIDS, malaria and other diseases	• Have halted by 2015 and begun to reverse the spread of HIV/AIDS • Achieve, by 2010, universal access to treatment for HIV/AIDS for all those who need it • Have halted by 2015 and begun to reverse the incidence of malaria and other major diseases
7.	Ensure environmental sustainability	• Integrate the principles of sustainable development into country policies and programmes and reverse the loss of environmental resources • Reduce biodiversity loss, achieving, by 2010, a significant reduction in the rate of loss • Halve, by 2015, the proportion of the population without sustainable access to safe drinking water and basic sanitation • Achieve, by 2020, a significant improvement in the lives of at least 100 million slum dwellers
8.	Develop a Global Partnership For Development	• Develop further an open, rule-based, predictable, non-discriminatory trading and financial system • Address the special needs of least developed countries • Address the special needs of landlocked developing countries and small island developing States • Deal comprehensively with the debt problems of developing countries • In cooperation with pharmaceutical companies, provide access to affordable essential drugs in developing countries • In cooperation with the private sector, make available benefits of new technologies, especially information and communications

Source: Millennium Development Goals. United Nations

While the element of environmental sustainability was included in the MDGs, the achievement of "core" development gains was the chief aim. The MDGs were notably successful in reducing poverty and hunger, and the element of environmental sustainability did not receive adequate profile under the MDGs. It was argued that they only placed symbolic emphasis on the environment, and several key dimensions related to environmental sustainability were not adequately represented. Missing perspectives included areas such as ocean acidification, ecosystem-based management and resilience. In addition, regional achievement of targets was uneven, and the poorest regions of the world achieved the least success in meeting individual targets pertaining to the environment[15]. In fact, as economic activity picked up pace in these regions, it generated adverse environmental externalities (e.g. increased use of wood for industrial purposes, more carbon emissions, etc.)[16].

As an example, and at the global level, the proportion of deforested land area decreased, but at a minimal rate, from 32% to 31% - with the fastest rate of deforestation experienced in sub-Saharan Africa, Latin America, Southeastern Asia and Oceania. Moreover, the quality of the remaining forest area was poor and characterized by reduced biodiversity. The level of carbon dioxide emissions from fossil fuels increased by over 40% between 1990 and 2010. While developed regions achieved a 4% decrease in carbon dioxide emissions, this was more than offset by a tripling of emissions in the rapidly developing regions of the world, such as Southeastern Asia. Data also showed that between 1990 and 2012, the percentage of species that were expected to become extinct in the near future increased slightly from 7.9% to 8.7% at the global level, leading to loss of biodiversity. While access to clean drinking water increased, gender and regional inequity remained. A large disparity between rural and urban settings also continued. Progress on improved access to sanitation facilities was also behind target in 2010[17].

In the wake of this realization, world governments galvanized the process to adopt a new set of global goals from 2015 to 2030, which placed equal emphasis on economic growth and sustainability. Thus, in the run up to Rio+20 summit in June 2012, a special global sustainability panel was appointed by the UN Secretary General, Ban Ki-Moon. This panel developed a set of Sustainable Development Goals (SDGs), which presented a general consensus on which the world would move into the future[18].

	Sustainable Development Goals
1.	End poverty in all its forms everywhere
2.	End hunger, achieve food security and improved nutrition and promote sustainable agriculture
3.	Ensure healthy lives and promote well-being for all at all ages
4.	Ensure inclusive and equitable quality education and promote lifelong learning opportunities for all
5.	Achieve gender equality and empower all women and girls
6.	Ensure availability and sustainable management of water and sanitation for all
7.	Ensure access to affordable, reliable, sustainable and modern energy for all
8.	Promote sustained, inclusive and sustainable economic growth, full and productive employment and decent work for all
9.	Build resilient infrastructure, promote inclusive and sustainable industrialization and foster innovation
10.	Reduce inequality within and among countries
11.	Make cities and human settlements inclusive, safe, resilient and sustainable
12.	Ensure sustainable consumption and production patterns
13.	Take urgent action to combat climate change and its impacts
14.	Conserve and sustainably use the oceans, seas and marine resources for sustainable development
15.	Protect, restore and promote sustainable use of terrestrial ecosystems, sustainably manage forests, combat desertification, and halt and reverse land degradation and halt biodiversity loss
16.	Promote peaceful and inclusive societies for sustainable development, provide access to justice for all and build effective, accountable and inclusive institutions at all levels
17.	Strengthen the means of implementation and revitalize the Global Partnership for Sustainable Development

Source: The Sustainable Development Goals Report. United Nations. 2017

The chief aim of these SDGs is to continue the momentum generated by the MDGs while also providing profile to efforts combating climate change and making development more sustainable[19]. At the heart of the SDGs lies the concept of the triple bottom line – the focus on people, profit, and planet - translating into the integration of the economy, the society and the environment. While the MDGs primarily proposed targets for poor countries, the SDGs are universal in nature. They identify goals and challenges that all the countries around the world need to address in order to achieve sustainability targets[20].

In addition, a number of international treaties and agreements for environmental protection have been signed by various countries. The United Nations Framework Convention on Climate Change (UNFCCC) is one such international environmental treaty that aims to stabilize and limit the amount of greenhouse gas in the earth's atmosphere to minimize anthropogenic interference with the climate system. 165 countries signed the treaty, but the treaty lacked binding limits on greenhouse gas emissions and enforcement mechanisms. The parties to the Convention (i.e. the signatory countries) have met once every year since 1995 at the annual Conference of the Parties (COP) to evaluate the progress made in tackling climate change.

In December 1997, the Kyoto Protocol was concluded as an extension of the Convention. The Kyoto Protocol is also an international treaty that specified legally binding emission reduction targets. However, the Kyoto Protocol is not universal, and was established on the principle of "common but differentiated responsibilities"[21]. It placed the onus of reducing greenhouse gas (GHG) emissions on developed countries on the grounds that they were historically responsible for the existing levels of greenhouse gases in the atmosphere owing to more than 150 years of industrial activity. The Kyoto Protocol entered into force on 17th February, 2005. The rules for the implementation of the Protocol were adopted at COP 7 in 2001 in Morocco, and came to be known as the 'Marrakesh Accords'. The commitment period for these Accords was between 2008 and 2012. During this commitment period, 37 industrialized countries and the European Community committed to reducing GHG emissions to an average of 5% against 1990 levels. In 2012, the second commitment period started in Qatar, and came to be known as the Doha Amendment. During this commitment period, parties were obliged to reduce GHG emissions by at least 18% below 1990 levels in between 2013 and 2020.

Following the Doha Amendment, the Paris Agreement was adopted at COP21 in 2015 to govern greenhouse gas emission reductions from 2020. The Paris Agreement's chief objective is to strengthen the global response to climate change by keeping global temperature rise below 2 degrees Celsius above pre-industrial levels and to pursue efforts to limit this increase to less than 1.5 degrees in this century. Moreover, the agreement also emphasizes supporting countries in dealing with the effects of climate change and global warming. Under the agreement, all parties are required to publicly outline their Nationally Determined Contributions, which comprise of the specific climate actions and steps they intend to take in their countries. Each country determines its own contributions in the context of national priorities, circumstances and capabilities[22].

These are all great global and national efforts, and all heading in the right direction. Naturally, the momentum is subject to political and economic pressures each nation faces. In 2017 the US President, Donald Trump, withdrew his country from the COP21 commitments. Some countries moved faster than others, while various forms of alliances and forums sprung up to drive the global efforts.

While these are top-down government-driven target setting and policy interventions, there is one key stakeholder that could potentially hold the key to successfully addressing the sustainability challenge, the private sector.

The role of the private sector

Businesses have the monopoly to create wealth and resources by generating a profit. Institutions from other sectors (civil society and public sector) can use these resources to undertake work for social wellbeing, but these sectors do not have the ability to create resources, since their raison d'etre is not profit-generation. Corporations and firms are the key players in generating economic activity (and consequently imposing environmental externalities), and they have the potential to initiate change and devise solutions that make economic growth more environmentally-friendly and sustainable. This started to happen many decades ago, with varying motivations and mixed results.

Overall, and while governments around the world were committing to create an eco-system that balances economic growth with environmental sustainability, the private sector has also played a prominent part in making business practices more sustainable.

As an example, let us look at the international climate agreements and how corporations supported those. Literature informs us that the stance of the business sector has changed drastically since the adoption of UNFCCC in 1992. In the early 1990s, the business sector (mostly in developed industrial nations) was not in favor of climate change regulations and undertook obstructive lobbying to prevent the formulation of climate change policies[23]. It was seen as "bad for business" and the science behind it was debatable. By the time the Kyoto Protocol took place, the global business sector was divided into two factions: fossil-fuel dependent sectors, and businesses that were placing their stakes on a low-carbon future (e.g. renewable future) or businesses that were faced with cost increases in the wake of climate change (e.g. insurance).

However, a gradual change was observed in the overall oppositional stance, and by the time the COP15 took place in Copenhagen in 2009, an increasing number of manufacturing and technology-based businesses were seen lending their support for restrictions on carbon emissions[24]. This was probably driven by more informed studies, increasing political pressure, and rising customer awareness and interest. By the time the Paris Agreement came into place, businesses were already welcoming a strong climate agreement. In fact, conferences for businesses were organized in parallel to the Paris negotiations, where several business leaders went to attend and speak at these events, and some even established voluntary alliances with the public sector and civil society (like the Global Alliance for Buildings and Construction – GABC – which works in association with the United Nations Environment Programme - UNEP).

In the United States alone, 81 large companies signed the American Business Act on Climate Pledge, demonstrating their support for the conclusion of the negotiations of the Paris Agreement in 2015. These companies (including Coca Cola, Facebook, IKEA USA, Kellogg's, McDonalds Corporation) had annual revenues exceeding US$ 3 trillion and a combined market capitalization of over US$ 5 trillion, and employed 9 million people[25].

This trend of corporate support for climate change policies is now gaining momentum due to several factors driving the shift in stance regarding climate change in the last two decades, namely customer preferences, political oversight, good citizenship, and business opportunities. Environmental sustainability is now starting to become a core element of business sustainability.

Firstly, awareness of climate risks is on the rise around the world, and in all corners of our societies, including the business world. Firms are increasingly realizing the risks and impact of climate change on business activity, and have started measuring and reporting their impact on the environment (including, for example, the emissions they produce), and the potential impact on that climate change has on the bottom line. A report issued by Citi GPS in 2015 revealed that not acting on climate change could potentially cost the global economy up to US$ 72 trillion by 2060[26]. In terms of individual enterprises, in 2014, Unilever's CEO Paul Polman reported that his company incurs a loss of more than US$ 300 million a year owing to natural disasters related to climate change[27], and Nike also voiced its concern over the heightened incidence of droughts in regions that produce the cotton that the company uses to manufacture sportswear[28].

Secondly, businesses have also started to realize the business and profit-maximization opportunities that carbon restrictions present. As the cost of solar energy declined around the world, it provided the push for investment in renewable energy. As a result, Chinese businesses jumped at the opportunity, positioning China as the global leader in solar energy production and installation[29]. Companies that were previously skeptical about going green on the grounds of cost hikes are now flocking to environmentally-friendly investments as a result of the recent sharp decline in cost of renewable energy and the price certainty that is associated with renewable energy. A recent report shows that clean energy measures undertaken by 190 Fortune 500 companies are saving them US$ 3.7 billion per annum, while also eliminating annual carbon pollution equivalent to 45 coal-fired power plants. As a result of these large savings, 63% of Fortune 100 companies have set one or more clean energy targets[30]. Amongst these Fortune 500 companies, 10% have set renewable energy targets, and almost half of those (including Walmart, Facebook, General Motors, Google, Apple) have committed to power 100% of their operations with renewable energy[31]. Sustainable practices have moved from simply caring for the environment to core operational imperatives and pure business decisions.

While profit maximization presents an important supply-side consideration for adopting eco-friendly solutions, the customer demand and advocacy for adopting these technologies is also a noteworthy factor driving this trend. Consumers are now demanding more sustainable practices from the businesses they deal with, and, in some sectors, rewarding such companies with their loyal business, or even premium payments. This trend is seen to be especially true when dealing with the next generation of millennials and Generation Z.

Communication technology and social media networks have enhanced the consciousness and awareness of the modern-day consumer and amplified the demand for transparency over corporate conduct. Irresponsible corporate conduct can come at the cost of expensive lawsuits, as well as loss of business reputation. A study conducted by Unilever reveals that a third of consumers (33%) are now choosing to buy from brands they believe are doing social or environmental good[32]. That is a huge shift, and those numbers will only grow as the awareness spreads.

The Edelman Trust Barometer 2017 shows that public trust in business has increased over the last three years (from 37% in 2014 to 52% in 2017), and is higher than public trust in governments (41%)[33]. This implies that public expectations from corporations to deliver and act in a sustainably responsible manner is also growing rapidly. This trend is confirmed in surveys exploring public expectations, which reveal that the majority of respondents believe that it is important for companies to minimize any negative impact they may have on the environment[34]. As a result, firms and corporations are moving beyond the mere pursuit of short term shareholders' economic interests. The new approach that successful businesses are adopting involves balancing value creation and improving the bottom-line, with managing the diverse and often, conflicting expectations of a growing spectrum of stakeholders (suppliers, employees, customers and the community at large). A difficult balance that aims to achieve a win-win outcome for the triple bottom line.

Creating shared value: the rise of collaborative governance

Legitimacy can be defined as a generalized perception or assumption that the actions of an entity are desirable, proper or appropriate within some socially constructed system of norms, values, beliefs and definitions[35]. To understand the trend of growing corporate legitimacy and accountability, one must understand the relationship between power and legitimacy. This is indeed an exciting and new lens with which to study the corporate world - one that is becoming more important in the age of social media, and informed and connected customers.

Traditionally, the concept of legitimacy has been consistently associated with the power of government. The state or government has various powers, and the monopolistic exertion of these powers maintains order in a Hobbesian world[36]. However, the possession of these powers presents to the government the problem of legitimacy, which is needed to justify the wielding of these powers. The government has to deliver against certain standards or promises in order to wield these powers in a legitimate manner.

This concept now is becoming more relevant, and more important, for corporate leaders. In today's world, businesses have the power to affect the lives of their stakeholders in important ways. They employ human resources, create livelihoods, generate economic value for investors, manage vital personal data, and have the ability to alter consumer perceptions with their products and services. Just like government power, corporate power can be abused by corporate leaders to work against the interest of shareholders, employees and consumers. Corporate scandals in the recent past (Enron, Tyco, Parmalat) are testimony to this abuse, and bring the concept of heightened corporate legitimacy to the forefront. In addition, several corporate environmental disasters of varying magnitude (Exxon oil spill, Bhopal gas tragedy, Volkswagen emissions scandal) have unfolded in the last few years, causing immense harm to the environment and the surrounding community.

In today's increasingly interconnected world, corporate legitimacy towards consumers takes center stage. With specific regard to the environment, the issue of greener and more eco-friendly policies is not only a responsible business decision, but one that will also be driven more and more by consumer preferences, especially in light of the changing demographics. The millennial generation, which will constitute half of the global workforce by 2020, expresses its opinions about environmental and social issues on social media. With these shifting demographics pointing to an increased emphasis on social responsibility and social media providing unfiltered and uncontrollable communications, companies must positively manage their sustainability practices to succeed. The impact of their actions (beyond the quality of their products and services) is defining - more and more - their legitimacy, and hence their future profitability and sustainability.

In the decades corresponding to the MDG's, one way companies have responded to the social concerns surrounding globalization and its social impact, was through their philanthropic activities. Corporate philanthropy is a company's efforts to donate money or resources to an organization or a cause, promoting and allowing employees to volunteer in the community, and/or the establishment or endorsement of charity foundations. Historically, companies have focused on contributing profits to causes that were important to their management (e.g. education). Some companies went further and set up foundations to address a wide range of social issues covering education, health, women empowerment, among others.

While these resources can be substantial, they tended to be isolated from the vision, mission and operation of the company, and -in some cases- its management and employees. More importantly, many multinational corporations started to recognize that philanthropic activity cannot replace the impact of the company doing business in a responsible and environmentally sustainable way, while measuring and reporting its impact on the societies it operates in and serves.

A step further from corporate philanthropy was the concept of Corporate Social Responsibility (CSR) where companies set social missions that considered different stakeholders when making a business decision. As a concept, CSR gained popularity across the corporations and international organizations. An industry grew around this and a wide range of companies started to focus on helping interested governments, corporations and individuals collaborated to further CSR objectives. Moreover, global and international organizations like OECD, ILO, and United Nations became prominent supporters of CSR activities, and have put in place frameworks and guidelines to catalyze CSR initiatives.

In 1979, Archie Carroll introduced his ideas about Corporate Social Responsibility and developed a CSR model with four categories of corporate responsibility organized from most to least important. In 1991, Carroll built further on this research and suggested that although the components are not mutually exclusive, the prioritization framework allows the manager to realize that the different types of obligations are in continuous conflict with each other. Analysis of this model identifies its consistent emphasis on economic and legal responsibilities, ethical and philanthropic elements having secondary importance. In Carroll's view, CSR is a relatively modest shift away from isolating philanthropy from the day-to-day company goals.[37]

A Multi-Dimensional CSR Prioritization Framework

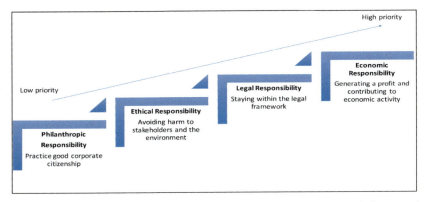

Source: The Pyramid of Corporate Social Responsibility: Toward the Moral Management of Organizational Stakeholders. Archie Carroll. Business Horizons. 34(4):39-48. July 1991.

Significant work was also undertaken to understand the factors that drive CSR within companies. In today's literature, and while there is no single leading argument for CSR, Simon Zadek[38] broke down the business case for CSR into four different categories:

(1) protect and defend company reputation
(2) justify benefits over costs
(3) integrate with company broader strategy
(4) learn, innovate and mitigate risk.

Thus, the business case for CSR was rooted in the desire of corporations to comply with community standards, be good corporate citizens, and improve public trust and their corporate reputation[39].

This was, by and large, a good thing and many positive outcomes were delivered. In the last decade, General Motors (GM)[40] has undertaken a number of initiatives to go green and improve environmental outcomes. In 2010, GM announced that Chevrolet – its largest brand and core product – will invest US$ 40 million in carbon offsetting projects in the United States. The potential impact of this initiative was the offsetting of 8 million metric tons of carbon dioxide emissions – the equivalent of emissions that came from the 1.9 million cars and trucks Chevrolet expected to sell in the same year. In the press release announcing this initiative, the company's CEO said, "Chevrolet's investment is an extension of the environmental initiatives we've been undertaking for years because the solution to global environmental challenges goes beyond just vehicles." In addition, GM's manufacturing facilities reduced their water usage on a per-vehicle basis by 32% between 2005 and 2010[41]. A conscious effort to reduce the use of fossil fuels at GM plants has also been made.

The business literature is full of similar stories and examples of successful CSR initiatives from corporations large and small, from all over the world. However, the more exciting shift was yet to come.

In the mid-2000s, a paradigm shift started taking shape and new concepts of corporate responsibility emerged. The most significant work in this regard was conducted by Michael Porter and Mark Kramer, who published an article in the Harvard Business Review discussing how corporate growth can be balanced with social welfare to create a win-win situation. They proposed the integration of CSR into corporate strategy, and leveraging CSR as a source of innovation and competitive advantage. The article called for a shift in the corporate perception of CSR – viewing it as a business opportunity, rather than treating it as a damage control measure or PR campaign.

They introduced a framework that businesses can use to[42]:

- identify the consequences of their actions on society
- explore opportunities to generate economic and social value
- determine which CSR initiatives to address and how.

The idea of Creating Shared Value (CSV) entered the business world and started taking shape.

Porter and Kramer argued that in an increasingly competitive corporate environment, businesses should continuously seek new ways to remain competitive without compromising on their social responsibility. Therefore, the challenge facing modern corporate managers was fulfilling the business's social obligations alongside its economic obligations. This marked a shift in the way businesses approached social responsibility[43] as the figure below shows.

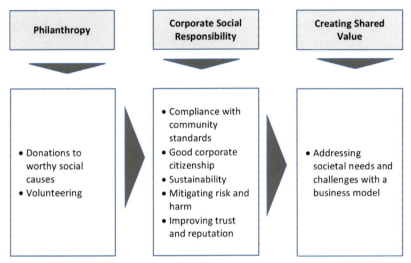

Source: *Creating Shared Value as Business Strategy. Michael E. Porter. Presentation for the Shared Value Leadership Summit Boston, MA. May 23rd, 2013*

Shared value creation is defined as policies and business practices that strengthen the competitiveness profile of a company, while also advancing the economic, environmental and social conditions in the communities it operates in. CSV called for the integration of social and environmental functions (and impacts) within the corporate strategy, where social and environmental concerns are not seen as disconnected challenges or problems – rather they are viewed as opportunities linked to business strategy.

While the concept makes theoretical sense, it is only when one sees it in practice that it starts to demonstrate its full potential for our societies.

Take Nestle as one example. Well known for some famous chocolate brands, Nestle is a large buyer of cocoa (414,000 tonnes of cocoa per annum, mainly for chocolate and confectionery but also for other products such as beverages). Faced with potential supply constraints for cocoa in 1999, Nestle developed the Nestle Cocoa Plan which would boost cocoa production and impact the way cocoa farming was done. Nestle's cocoa supplies come from major cocoa-growing countries including Côte d'Ivoire, Ghana, Brazil, Ecuador, Venezuela, Mexico and Indonesia. The majority of cocoa producers are small farmers with low productivity and incomes, living in poor communities, with depleted soils and older, less productive trees. They often resort to using their children for tasks that could be harmful to their physical or mental development and are therefore classified as child labour, and women in the cocoa supply chain are often under-rewarded for their work.

The Nestle Cocoa Plan aimed to improve the lives of farmers in the company's cocoa supply chain, based on the following pillars:

- Better farming, addressing issues such as agricultural practices and rejuvenation of plantations;
- Better lives, which seeks to empower women and eliminate child labour; and
- Better cocoa, which covers certification and building long-term relationships in the supply chain.

In 2016, 57,000 farmers were trained in improving yields, reducing cocoa diseases, and improving bean quality. Moreover, 2,160,000 new cocoa plants were sown to replace the old trees with low yield. It has also educated 35,000 community members and more than 12,000 farmers on child labour issues in Côte d'Ivoire. A Child Labour Monitoring and Remediation System (CLMRS) has been rolled out to help children get out of child labour. Schools were also set up to educate the children of the cocoa farming community. The company also supports women to carry out income-generating activities. It also set up a research and development center in Abidjan, and has built an upcountry experimental farm and training center. As a result of these efforts, the volume of Nestle Cocoa Plan cocoa stands at 140,933 tons, representing 34% of the total cocoa used by Nestle[44.] Nestle is doing well by doing good.

With more and more examples like these, CSV emerged as a more evolved extension of CSR, highlighting the shift from taking away profits to solve social and environmental challenges to a more strategic approach of generating economic value (i.e. profit) from activities that solve societal problems. Moreover, successful examples of shared value creating exposed businesses to new customer needs, new available markets, new value chain choices, and new ways to address external constraints – all of which are key elements of a successful business strategy.

Doing CSV right became a key part of doing business right for many leading firms, and the approach even helped many businesses identify new potential sources of competitive advantage. These businesses maintain that incorporating social dimensions into the value proposition enables cost reductions and presents opportunities for product differentiation[45].

A great example here is CVS Health, a leading American drugstore. CVS Health redefined its value proposition to improve health outcomes. In 2014, CVS became the first pharmacy to stop selling tobacco products in thousands of stores all over the country. The immediate short-term tradeoff in that decision was the loss of US$ 2 billion in annual revenue. However, the company began to see new customers in the stores, and more health plans and employers interested in choosing the pharmacy benefit management side of the business. CVS Health's goodwill among customers, healthcare providers, non-profits, and elected leaders improved. Moreover, following the decision to quit selling tobacco products, customers also suggested adding healthy foods to the CVS product mix. CVS followed this advice and introduced new and healthy products which were displayed at the front of the CVS store, while unhealthy food items were moved to the back. This was a profitable decision, as healthy alternatives sold well. CVS also operates a network of in-store clinics as an alternative to a doctor's office visit, which has expanded the role of pharmacists and nurse practitioners employed by CVS. Thus, CVS has had a marked transition in its corporate vision from improving the quality of human life to facilitating people's transition to better health.[46]

Therefore, the adoption of a CSV approach directs companies towards creating new ways of achieving positive economic outcomes, focusing on the right kind of net profits: profits that generate positive social externalities and solve societal problems rather than diminishing them[47].

Another great example here is Danone, a world leading food company. Danone realized that it had drifted away from its origins as maker of healthy foods. Therefore, in 2005, Danone decided to sell its beer, meat, and cheese business units and turned its focus back on water and dairy products. The company acquired new businesses in medical nutrition and baby foods. It created Innovation Committees within each business unit to provide healthy food for the maximum number of people. In 2013, Danone developed NutriPlanet, a database that gathers dietary, nutrition and health data in different cultures and communities. The idea behind developing this database was to understand country-specific cultural and food contexts and develop tailored products adapted to local issues [48]. These moves were pure business strategy for Danone, but also had many positive outcomes on public health, awareness, and offerings.

The concept of shared value is closely tied to the Blue Ocean strategy approach, in that businesses identify initiatives that are tied to the core business, but introduce an element of competition based on innovation. To create shared value, businesses have to think strategically, look for uncontested market spaces, and extend themselves from "competing to be the best" to "competing to be unique"[49]. Thus, the identification of a unique competitive position, which also has social and environmental benefits, lies at the heart of the concept of CSV.

On the supply side of this CSV equation, another driving force was in play. Governments have been going through an "era of austerity" for the past decade in the aftermath of the financial crisis of 2007-2008, and volatile commodity prices[50]. In the wake of tightening fiscal budgets, "affordable government" that can "do more with less" has become the order of the day. To navigate this rather complex and uncharted territory, governments are looking to collaborate with other sectors - namely business and civil society – to meet citizen expectations. This attempt at collaboration is aimed at breaking the silos and delivering sustainability outcomes that no single organization or sector has the knowledge or resources to achieve on its own.

For example, and according to UN Environment Program (UNEP) estimates, the cost of adapting to climate change for developing countries can potentially escalate to US$ 280 - US$ 500 billion per annum in the run up to 2050. While bilateral and multilateral funding to developing countries has increased in the last ten years, the "adaptation finance gap" is wide and likely to become wider in the coming years. The capacity of developing country governments (that have scarce resources) to generate the required finance is limited, and they will need to seek additional and innovative funding sources to meet this end [51].

Realizing these complex realities, the number of partnerships to address sustainability have grown exponentially in the last 15 years around the world. Governments are increasingly looking towards business for financial resources and competencies (such as innovation) that lie beyond the scope of public sector agencies. As a result, a new modus operandi – namely collaborative governance – is emerging, allowing the government to use external institutions and resources to coordinate and undertake collective effort. Collaborative governance is particularly valuable in natural resource management, as the degree of interconnectedness amongst stakeholders is very high [52].

Above and beyond the business sector's financial muscle, collaborative governance can enable governments to improve technical capacity, particularly in terms of data and information management processes. The co-management approach that is a principle tenet of collaborative governance, also fosters knowledge transfer and encourages innovation among government agencies [53].

Businesses and corporations are also the source of new eco-friendly technologies and adaptation services (e.g. weather observation technologies, early warning systems, etc.). Partnering with these firms to introduce these products and technologies is likely to be a far more economical option for governments [54]. Arguments about business having deeper insight into people's preferences are also made to support greater collaboration. Proponents argue that businesses understand citizen needs and preferences well, and – in some cases - better than their own governments, as they depend on this information to stay relevant and succeed on a day-to-day basis[55].

For businesses, collaborative governance promises improved reputation and corporate image, and an enhancement of critical competencies as businesses acquire new knowledge about existing problems. It can also allow businesses to identify previously unknown problems, as well as opportunities for developing new products and markets to address them [56]. Needless to say, collaboration also allows businesses to get closer to policymaking, and influence the discourse. They can lobby for policies that enhance certainty for low-carbon investments, and incentives for the development of pro-environment technologies and products.

The role of government in collaborative governance

Collaborative governance is, by definition, a two-way effort. While businesses have to adopt and learn new ways and paradigms, so do governments. To engage businesses in an effort to enhance sustainability and protect our environment, governments have many levers.

Key amongst these levers is the government's ability to help the private sector in scaling up existing capacity. Businesses, both big and small, are investing in sustainability efforts, but the means vary from firm to firm. Some are developing adaptation products and low-carbon solutions, while others are safeguarding their supply chains against climate change and the associated natural disasters. Government can play a key role here to scale up investments with high potential, and ensure that the solutions reach the most vulnerable parts of the population. Specific measures that governments can take in this area are awareness raising, provision of technical assistance, granting of concessional loans and tax breaks and/or credits, and giving subsidies and/or grants. For example, companies working to address adaptation in high-risk sectors like agriculture should be identified, and the community should be enabled (e.g. through awareness raising and vouchers for procuring the company's products) to purchase their products. In this scenario, the government plays the role of a pulling force, increasing the market demand for adaptation products and green technology by increasing benefits to the end-users[57].

Another area that the government can have a major impact on is correcting market failures. The majority of businesses are already taking measures to protect themselves against adverse environmental changes. Nevertheless, some private firms (especially small and medium enterprises) are reluctant to invest in adaptation efforts owing to the cost or risk involved. This is a case of a good that has the potential for generating a positive externality, but is being under-produced or under-consumed. In this regard, governments can correct market failures through several ways, mainly policies and initiatives that indirectly strengthen resilience among vulnerable groups and generate demand for adaptation products. They can use "push" instruments that reduce the cost of technologies and products for businesses, and mitigate the risks of technology innovation. Tax breaks, low-interest loans, and capacity building activities can be used to encourage these businesses to invest in eco-friendly products and technologies.

There are many examples of such initiatives. In France, OSEO public investment bank offers loans at favorable rates and without collateral from EUR 50,000 to EUR 3 million for up to seven years for SMEs who adopt environmentally friendly technologies (with the share of capital costs exceeding 60%) or develop new ones[58], while in the UK the Energy Saving Trust (a UK-wide non-profit organization) provides zero- interest small business loans of up to GBP 100,000 to help businesses install renewable energy technologies or measures that reduce energy consumption.

Public incubators and competitions for small businesses can also be introduced to stimulate the development of adaptation products and technologies. Governments can also put standards (e.g. climate-resistant building standards) and regulations in place to ensure that businesses invest in critical adaptation areas. The impact of these corrective policies and regulations will vary from business to business, depending on its size, level of maturity and the industry/sector it belongs to. [59]

Last, but by no means least, governments can, and should, encourage public-private-partnerships (PPPs) in the sustainability domain. Irrespective of its social value, the private sector is unlikely to invest in producing a product or service that does not create economic value, i.e. profit. As a result, the private sector will not invest in a public good (e.g. water infrastructure, flood protection, disaster management, etc.), as this would not be a profit-making venture. Consequently, governments have to invest in public goods and services. However, the private sector can be engaged through a public-private partnership (PPP) to design, construct, upgrade, implement or manage a government-sponsored project. These are contractual agreements between a business and a government agency to combine the capabilities and assets of each sector to co-produce public services. Under a PPP agreement, both parties agree to share risks and rewards of the project according to a pre-set formula.

In China, with the rapid growth of population and urbanization, the amount of Municipal Solid Waste (MSW) generated has skyrocketed. In 2004, cities in the country produced 190 million tons of MSW, which included residential, institutional, commercial, street cleaning, and non-treated waste from industries. The majority of MSW is disposed by landfill (both sanitary and uncontrolled) and to a smaller extent, by incineration and composting. The city of Wenzhou, in China's Zhejiang Province, was generating circa 400,000 tons of household waste per annum. The volume of waste was increasing at the rate of 8-10% every year, and it was disposed into two landfills run by the City government. In 2002, the local government established a Build-Operate-Transfer (BOT) partnership with Wei Ming Environmental Protection

Engineering – a local private contractor. The agreement was that Wei Ming would invest in the building and operating of a new MSW-to-energy incinerator plant for 25 years. The ownership of the plant would revert to government at the end of the agreement period without any additional compensation to Wei Ming. The incinerator plant has a design capacity of 320 tons of MSW per day and electricity generation of up to 25 million kilowatts annually. The first phase of the plant would be able to treat 160 tons per day. This would allow the plant to generate 9 million kWh a year, of which 7 million kWh would be available for sale. The plant would also receive a service fee from the Wenzhou city government for the disposal of MSW at a rate of CNY 73.8 per ton. The implementation of the plant is in line with the objectives of China's Renewable Energy Law passed in 2005. It is supported through a range of preferential policies and government incentives, including the requirement that electricity network operators purchase electricity generated by qualified energy producers using renewable energy sources. The project also enjoyed an exemption from corporate income tax for the first five years and immediate refund of value-added tax. In addition, the electricity generated through the project was sold at the higher tariff reserved for energy from renewable sources[60].

Clearly, a well-structured public-private partnership can allow the two sectors to leverage each other's complementary strengths. These partnerships can enable the public sector to use the intellectual capital of the private sector to operate a sustainability initiative in a more effective and efficient manner. Similarly, the private sector may have the technical know-how, but it has to rely on the government to generate the appropriate incentives and opportunities for innovation[61]. In 1999, the Woking Borough Council - a public authority based outside of London - established Thameswey Energy Limited as an Energy Service Company (ESCo) that owns, operates, and manages the heat, electricity, and water supply in the borough. Thameswey is a PPP between the Borough Council and Xergi Limited, a Danish energy company which owns 10% of the shares. The PPP model allowed Woking to surpass government controls on local government spending, establish a Combined Heat and Power (CHP) plant, and build a private wire renewable energy system and fuel cell CHP system. The private system also allows the Borough to save on fees associated with accessing the national power grid, to which it is connected as a back-up supplier. Between 1990 and 2004, the Borough experienced a 48.6% reduction in energy consumption and a 17.23% reduction in CO_2 emissions from 2002. Moreover, the free or subsidized insulation that all residents received allowed the Borough to save 91,270 tonnes of energy per year. According to the Borough, the main reasons for the project's success was the technical, financial, and commercial innovation gained by working in partnership with the private sector. The project also demonstrates how a PPP model can offer additional flexibility and capital even in a stringent planning environment[62].

Irrespective of which mechanism is adopted, it is clear that the synergy between the government and the private sector is likely to generate positive sustainability outcomes. Each sector can play on the strengths of the other, and contribute its own to create a climate-resilient society. Given the challenges and constraints facing governments today, there is a strong case for businesses to share the burden of creating a liveable world for this generation and the next.

(Endnotes)

1. Sustainability – A Systems Approach. Anthony M H Clayton & Nicholas J Radcliffe. Earthscan Publications Limited, London. 1997
2. Preindustrial Human Impacts on Global and Regional Environment. Christopher E Doughty. Annual Review of Environment and Resources. Vol. 38:503-527. 2013
3. The 4th Industrial Revolution. Klaus Schwab. World Economic Forum. 2016
4. Silent Spring (40th Anniversary Edition). Rachel Carson. Houghton Mifflin Company, New York. 2002
5. The Ecological Impact of the Industrial Revolution. Eric McLamb. HYPERLINK http://www.ecology.com/2011/09/18/ecological-impact-industria http://www.ecology.com/2011/09/18/ecological-impact-industrial-revolution/. 2011
6. Sustainable Development Goals for a New Era. Jeffrey D. Sachs. Horizons, No. 1. Autumn 2014
7. The Fourth Industrial Revolution. Klaus Schwab. World Economic Forum. 2015
8. This is according to the United Nation's Official definition of extreme poverty
9. The state of the poor: where are the poor, where is extreme poverty harder to end, and what is the current profile of the world's poor? World Bank. 2013
10. Living Planet Report. World Wildlife Fund. 2012
11. Living Planet Report. World Wildlife Fund. 2012
12. The Anthropocene. Paul. J. Crutzen. In: Ehlers E., Krafft T. (eds) Earth System Science in the Anthropocene. Springer, Berlin, Heidelberg. 2006
13. Sustainable Development Goals for a New Era. Jeffrey D. Sachs. Horizons, No. 1. Autumn 2014
14. Planetary boundaries: Exploring the safe operating space for humanity. Johan Rockstrom et al. Ecology and Society 14(2): 32. 2009
15. Global Goals and the Environment: Progress and prospects. International Institute for Sustainable Development. 2015.
16. The Millennium Development Goals and Climate Change: Taking Stock and Looking Ahead. German Watch. 2010.
17. Global Goals and the Environment: Progress and prospects. International Institute for Sustainable Development. 2015.

18. From Millennium Development Goals to Sustainable Development Goals. Jeffrey D. Sachs. Lancet; 379: 2206–11. 2012
19. From MDGs to SDGs. Sustainable Development Goals Fund. HYPERLINK http://w/ http://w ww.sdgfund.org/mdgs-sdgs. 2017.
20. 20 From Millenniu m Development Goa ls to Susta inable Development Goals. Jeffrey D. Sachs. Lancet; 379: 2206–11. 2012
21. Kyoto Protocol to the United Nations Framework Convention on Climate Change. United Nations Framework Convention on Climate Change. 1998
22. What is an INDC?. World Resources Institute. http://www.wri. org/indc-definition
23. Intense Lobbying Against Global Warming Treaty. The New York Times. HYPERLINK http://www.nytimes.com/1997/12/07/us/intense-lobbyin http://www.nytimes.com/1997/12/07/us/intense-lobbyin g-against-global-warming-treaty.html?mcubz=0. 1997
24. Business involvement in climate negotiations has come a long way. LSE Business Review. 2015
25. 81 Companies sign American Business Act on Climate Change Pledge. Biofuels Digest. HYPERLINK http://w/ http://w w w.biofuelsdigest.com/bdiges t/2015/10/25/81-companies-sign-american-business-act-on-c limate-change-pledge/. 2015
26. Energy Darwinism II- Why a low carbon future doesn't have to cost the Earth. Citi GPS. 2015
27. UNILEVER CEO: We Need To Do More To Fight Climate Change. Business Insider. HYPERLINK http://w/ http://w w w.businessinsider.com/unilever-ce o-speaks-on-climate-change-2014 -12. 2014
28. Industry Awakens to Threat of Climate Change. The New York Times. https:// HYPERLINK http://www.nytimes.com/2014/01/24/science/earth/threa www.nytimes.com/2014/01/24/science/earth/threat-to-bottom-line-spur s-action-on-climate.html. 2014
29. China's solar power capacity more than doubles in 2016. Reuters. HYPERLINK http://w/ http://w ww.reuters.com/article/us-china-solar-idUSKBN15J0G7. 2017
30. Power Forward 3.0: How the largest US companies are capturing business value while addressing climate change. World Wildlife Fund, Calvert Investments, CDP and Ceres. 2017
31. Power Forward 3.0: How the largest US companies are capturing business value while addressing climate change. World Wildlife Fund, Calvert Investments, CDP and Ceres. 2017
32. Report shows a third of consumers prefer sustainable brands. Unilever. https://w w w.unilever.com/news/press-releases/2017/ report-shows-a-thir d-of-consumers-prefer-sustainable-brands. html. 2017

33 Edelman Trust Barometer 2017. Edelman. http://www.edelman.com/executive-summary/. 2017
34 High Expectations for Corporate Behavior. Public Affairs Pulse Survey 2015. https://pac.org/pulse/?p=486. 2015
35 Managing Legitimacy: Strategic and Institutional Approaches. Mark C. Suchman. The Academy of Management Review Vol. 20, No. 3. July, 1995
36 Legitimacy and Corporate Governance. Cary Coglianese. Faculty Scholarship - Paper 145. 2007
37 The Pyramid of Corporate Social Responsibility: Toward the Moral Management of Organizational Stakeholders. Archie Carroll. Business Horizons. 34(4):39-48. July 1991.
38 Doing Good and Doing Well: Making the Business Case for Corporate Citizenship. Simon Zadek. Research Report 1282-00- RR. The Conference Board, New York. 2000
39 Creating shared value. Michael E. Porter & Mark R. Kramer. Harvard Business Review. January-February 2011.
40 The Case of GM's CSR Initiative: Why Good Intentions Are Not Enough. Environmental Leader. ht t ps://w w w.env iron- me nt a l le a d e r.c om /2 011/01/t he- c a se- of- g ms- c sr-i n itiativ e-why-good-intentions-are-not-enough/. 2011
41 Resource Preservation Fact Sheet. General Motors. https:// HYPERLINK http://www/ www.gm.com/content/dam/gm/en us/english/Group3/sustainability/sustainabilitypdf/GM Resource Preservation Fact Sheet.pdf. 2015
42 Strategy & Society: The Link between Competitive Advantage and Corporate Social Responsibility. Michael E. Porter & Mark. R. Kramer. Harvard Business Review.;84(12):78-92, 163. Dec 2006
43 Creating Shared Value as Business Strategy. Michael E. Porter. Presentation for the Shared Value Leadership Summit Boston, MA. May 23rd, 2013
44 Nestle Cocoa Plan. Nestle. HYPERLINK http://www.nestle.com/csv/commu- http://www.nestle.com/csv/commu- nities/nestle-cocoa-plan. 2016.
45 Creating Shared Value as Business Strategy. Michael E. Porter. Presentation for the Shared Value Leadership Summit Boston, MA. May 23rd, 2013
46 At CVS, Improving Health Is Just Good Business - An interview with Helena B. Foulkes Shared Value Initiative. https://shared- value.org/g roups/cvs-improving-health-just-good-business. 2016
47 Creating Shared Value: A Paradigm Shift from Corporate Social Responsibility to Creating Shared Value. Bolanle Deborah Motilewa, E.K. Rowland Worlu, Gbenga Mayowa Agboola, Marvellous Aghogho Chidinma Gberevbie. International Journal of Social, Behavioral, Educational, Economic, Business and Industrial Engineering, 10(8). 2016

48 NutriPlanet: Using Big Data to Boost Nutrition. Charlotte Sarrat. Danone Nutricia Research. HYPERLINK http://nutrijournal.danone.com/en/ http://nutrijournal.danone.com/en/articles/stories/nutriplanet-using-big-data-to-boost-nutrition/. 2013
49 Blue Ocean Strategy: How To Create Uncontested Market Space And Make The Competition Irrelevant. W. Chan Kim & Renee Mauborgne. Harvard Business Review Press, Cambridge, MA. 2005
50 The Future of Government. PriceWaterhouse Coopers. 2013
51 The Adaptation Gap Report. UN Environment. 2016
52 Collaborating: Finding Common Ground for Multiparty Problems. Barbara Gray. Jossey-Bass, San Francisco.
53 Overcoming locally based collaboration constraints. Richard D. Margerum. Society & Natural Resources, 20(2): 135–152. 2007.
54 Why We Must Engage the Private Sector in Climate Change Adaptation Efforts. Alan Miller for the World Bank Blog. http:// blogs.worldbank.org/climatechange/why-we-must-engage-private-sector-climate-change-adaptation-efforts. 2014
55 Who is leading action on climate change - the Private Sector or Government? Jonathan Shopley. Natural Capital Partners. https:// HYPERLINK http://www.naturalcapitalpartners.com/news-media/post/who-is-leadin www.naturalcapitalpartners.com/news-media/post/who-is-leading-action-on-climate-change-the-private-sector-or-government. 2016
56 Sustainabiliy Through Partnerships: Capitalizing on Collaboration. Network for Business Sustainability. 2013
57 'New' instruments of environmental governance: Patterns and pathways of change. Andrew Jordan, Rüdiger K.W. Wurzel & Anthony R. Zito. Environ. Politics, 12, 1–24. 2003
58 Environmental Policy Toolkit for Greening SMEs in EU Eastern Partnership countries. EaPGreen. 2015
59 3 Ways Governments Can Involve the Private Sector in Climate Change Adaptation. World Resources Institute. 2013
60 Municipal Solid Waste treatment: Case Study of Public–Private Partnerships (PPPs) in Wenzhou. World Bank. HYPERLINK http://ppp.world-/ http://ppp.world-bank.org/public-private-partnership/sites/ppp.worldbank.org/files/ppp testdumb/documents/urbandev-prc-nov2010-waste. pdf. 2010.
61 5 public-private partnerships pushing the sustainability envelope. Mike Hower. GreenBiz. https://www.greenbiz.com/article/5-public-private-partnerships-pushing-sustainability-envelope. 2015
62 Public-Private Partnerships in Sustainable Urban Development. Urban Land Institute. 2011.

Chapter 2

Business and the society: quantifying the impact

What can be measured, can be managed[63]

Traditionally, businesses have focused their energies on measuring and enhancing their economic success. However, global economic shifts over the past few decades have generated a new normal characterized by more volatile economic growth[64] and technological disruption. The business environment today is going through a structural transformation driven by disruptive technology and the rise of data, shifting values and new digital generations, and increasing concerns about climate change.

Stakeholder concern regarding the impact of climate change is increasing. Renewed vigor related to tackling climate change and halting global warming was witnessed at the COP23 in Paris in November 2017. While the withdrawal of the United States from the Paris agreement dampened hope for the fight against climate change, business groups, civil society organizations, and some American cities attended COP23 and pledged to honor the Paris deal irrespective of the government's stance. Former New York City mayor Michael Bloomberg has committed to pay the US$ 15 million in UNFCCC administration costs if the US government does not. A report detailing the scope and scale of non-federal climate change action in the US was also presented to the UNFCCC Executive Secretary Patricia Espinosa.

The World Economic Forum's Global Risks Report surveys almost 1000 global experts and decision-makers about the most significant risks facing the world. According to the 2018 report, four of the five high-impact risks facing the world are environmental, and the probability of their occurrence is higher than average. These include extreme weather events, natural disasters, failure of climate change mitigation and adaptation, and water crises. Extreme weather incurred massive human and economic costs in 2017. In the US, seventeen named storms including Harvey and Irma, caused $200 billion worth of damages.[65]

Furthermore, monsoon flooding in the Subcontinent took over 1200 lives and affected more than 40 million people.[66] In the wake of these crises, the environment and climate change have been key focus areas of the World Economic Forum in Davos in the last few years.

Similarly, climate change was also prioritized as a key agenda item for the G20 Presidency in 2017. A policy document pertaining to environmental damage was also developed to outline the priorities of the summit. This document placed emphasis on boosting technological innovation and investing in future-oriented industries. A common G20 framework linking climate and energy policy and creating a reliable investment climate to better manage environmental risks was also highlighted.[67]

In addition, a survey released a week before the G7 summit in May 2017, revealed that 84% of the respondents considered climate change to be a "global catastrophic risk." The survey, which polled 8000 people in eight countries – the United States, China, India, Britain, Australia, Brazil, South Africa and Germany – indicates that people now view climate change to be a more significant threat than other traditional or rising concerns such as population growth, use of weapons of mass destruction, and spread of epidemics.[68] A similar analysis was presented in the Global Catastrophic Risks report, produced jointly in 2016 by the Global Challenges Foundation, the Future of Humanity Institute (FHI) and the Global Priorities Project at Oxford University in the United Kingdom. This report identified climate change to be an anthropogenic risk, which could trigger a range of global challenges including environmental degradation, migration, and the possibility of resource conflict. According to the report, the habitability of the planet can also be endangered if global warming exceeds 6°C. While the likelihood of this is low, it is nevertheless a realistic possibility if GHG emissions are not cut sufficiently, or if the sensitivity of the climate system is different from what is expected, or strong positive feedback loops in the carbon cycle.[69]

As more and more research emerges on the topic, stakeholders have started directing their resources and energies towards tackling climate change in their own respective capacities. In the development space, donor agencies have started prioritizing the environment by supporting initiatives that tackle environmental health risks, especially in developing countries. According to World Bank estimates, approximately 12.6 million people lose their lives every year due to environmental health risks. In response to this, between 2009 and 2016, World Bank commitments for environmental health and pollution management amounted to US$ 7 billion. Moreover, in 2014, the World Bank established a Multi-Donor Trust Fund for Pollution Management and Environmental Health to promote targeted measures to tackle air pollution in selected low income countries including China, Egypt, India, Nigeria, South Africa and Vietnam.[70]

Increasing consumer awareness about sustainability and environmental issues is another trend that is gaining momentum. Products and services produced by companies who have established a reputation for environmental stewardship are more attractive to today's youngest consumers.[71] Studies show that despite the tough economic climate in the last few decades, the majority of millennials are willing to pay more for sustainable consumer offerings. A Nielsen survey shows that 8 out of 10 millennials correlate their buying decision to the responsible efforts the producer or retailer is making. The study also shows that 73% of millennials are willing to try a new or unfamiliar product if it supports a good cause.[72]

This has important implications for businesses, as millennials constitute an influential and fast-growing consumer market. In the US alone, there are over 92 million millennials spending approximately US$ 600 billion every year.[73] In the wake of this changing consumer landscape, companies and retailers are being compelled to adopt more sustainable and environmentally approaches to make their products more attractive to this new generation of buyers.

Thus, it is clear that in this altered business landscape, shareholder preferences are not the only determining factors influencing the business decision-making process. They expect businesses to be more transparent and adhere to higher standards of responsibility, accountability and openness[74]. They expect companies to report the impact of their engagements on the environment, the local society, and our overall supply chain and ecosystem they operate in. As a result, businesses had to extend beyond the narrow measurement of financial performance and economic impact, and started assessing their contribution in the socio-economic and environmental spheres as well. In a span of less than three decades, the corporate world has moved from merely reporting financials to a wide array of impact measures.

Understanding and managing environmental impact is good for business

It is important to keep in mind that the adoption of the environmental lens for impact measurement is not only a demand-driven phenomenon. Businesses might have started doing this type of measurement and reporting as part of wider, and growing, awareness of the issue from stakeholders (governments, consumers, etc.) but they also see business implications.

Today, many companies are fully aware of the natural drivers of the so-called Green Wave, and the extent to which environmental issues can jeopardize supply chains and limit growth. In order to mitigate the risks that climate change poses to their potential to conduct business and grow, companies are having to rethink their strategies with an eye on environmental impacts and regulatory constraints. As early as the mid-1990s, businesses started realizing that supply chain constraints caused by climate change can trigger severe bottlenecks for production. An example of this is Unilever, which realized that supply for the frozen fish sticks business would be unreliable as the world's oceans run out of fish owing to overfishing. To combat this challenge, Unilever partnered with World Wildlife Fund to establish the Marine Stewardship Council. The Council was an autonomous body to promote sustainable fisheries around the world to protect the aquatic environment. To ensure a continuous stock of fish, the Council certified fisheries which adhered to total catch limits. In 2005, Unilever committed to buying all its fish from sustainable sources.[75]

Corporations are trying to manage downside risks posed by climate change, and some are even profiting from the new market opportunities that are emerging. For example, over the last few years, GE has invested billions of dollars in acquiring and developing its water infrastructure business. GE's ZeeWeed membrane technology is the basis for its membrane bioreactor (MBR) systems that use ultrafiltration membranes to produce the highest quality of water for reuse. These MBR plants are being widely deployed around the world for municipal and industrial plants to treat wastewater.[76] These investments have enabled GE to position itself as a leading solution provider for recycling and reusing water for industrial, irrigation, municipal and drinking water needs.[77]

Philips is another example of a company riding the clean-tech wave while also improving its bottomline. As the producer of one in four of the world's lights, in 2009, Philips invested roughly US$ 5 billion in light-emitting diodes or LED technology.[78] LED technology is more energy efficient and LED lights have a longer life than their conventional counterparts. Since then, Philips has integrated LED lights as a mainstream product and has also built on the LED technology to facilitate the development of a web-based street lighting management system that helps address the challenge of urbanization and the resulting pressure on energy.[79]

There is also a business case for environmental thinking and monitoring how a business affects the natural environment. This strategic focus is becoming more and more mainstream in strategic planning. A UNDP and GRI report released in 2016 reveals that 44% of the companies surveyed measured environmental impact in order to inform strategy and operations, while only 9% of companies measured impact for the sole purpose of meeting stakeholder expectations (client requirements and regulatory/policy requirements).[80]

In what they describe as the transition from green to gold, Esty and Winston argue that the environmental lens is a useful strategy tool that companies can leverage to improve corporate innovation and build competitive advantage.[81] Companies are increasingly realizing the top-line potential of growth opportunities that the Green Wave offers. They are incorporating an eco-advantage mindset to design and sharpen their business strategies. These WaveRiders are not only cutting operational costs and reducing environmental expenses, but are also identifying and reducing environmental and regulatory risks in their operations. But most importantly, these companies are finding ways to generate revenues by designing and marketing products that are eco-friendly and meet customer expectations of sustainability.[82]

However, this eco-advantage mindset does not come naturally. In fact, it has to be fostered and harnessed using specific tools that can help companies step up to challenges and recognize opportunities for further growth. Esty and Winston refer to this process of thinking and analyzing as Eco-Tracking, which enables companies to answer questions that are fundamental, but often unfamiliar. For example, businesses need to understand what their greatest environmental impacts are, and how and where in the supply chain these impacts arise. It is equally important for companies to analyze how they are viewed in terms of their environmental performance – by peers as well as customers and suppliers.[83] Therefore, businesses have to make a conscious and concerted effort to minimize their environmental costs, leverage new market opportunities, and become a force for good by driving environmental concerns at the heart of their business strategies.[84]

- The potential for upside benefits: The proverbial "gold" that smart businesses can extract from going green includes higher revenues, lower operational costs and even lower lending rates from banks that see reduced risk in companies with carefully constructed environmental-management systems. In addition, impact measurement can strengthen decision-making and innovation, and enable companies to go from "green to gold"[85]. Companies can identify customer needs and design breakthrough products for a new eco-defined market, which can enhance profits and sustain shareholder value. To ride the Green Wave and simultaneously improve their bottom line, companies must identify the environmental needs of their customers and seize eco-advantage through breakthrough products and green marketing, while also paying attention to their costs.

Basic Rules to Build the Upside

• Look at the forest, not the trees - WaveRiders consider broad timeframes involved in investment and strategic decisions. Their calculations take into account the complete range of potential pay-offs including intangible gains, which take time to realize and are hard to quantify. They also analyze how value can be added across the full chain of production.
• Start at the top – Commitment and willingness of their leadership to incorporate environmental sustainability into all business strategies and plans is essential for all WaveRiders.
• "No" is not an option – Setting ambitious goals and targets, and refusing to accept failure is integral for the management of companies that want to leverage Eco-Advantage.
• Take perception into account – WaveRiders understand that their reputation and stakeholder perception about their environmental performance is vital and must be considered for all key decisions.
• Do the right thing – Core values are important determinants of corporate decisions, and these values must be upheld even if immediate gains are not obvious.

Source: Green to gold: how smart companies use environmental strategy to innovate, create value, and build competitive advantage. Daniel Esty and Andrew Winston. Hoboken, NJ: John Wiley & Sons. 2009

An example of this can be found in Toyota's decision to produce and market its energy efficient hybrid car called Prius. In an environment where the track record of electric vehicles was poor, Toyota executives saw potential in introducing a hybrid vehicle. In 2004, Prius became the Car of the Year, and Toyota was raising prices and expanding production, while other car manufacturers in the US were struggling to survive. Toyota has since integrated sustainability into its broad strategy, and has valued innovation, and has been working to make its cars more energy efficient and smarter.[86]

Similarly, green marketing can increase sales by building a product's position and enhancing customer loyalty on the green qualities of the product. To illustrate, Wausau Paper – an American pulp and paper company – launched a new eco-friendly brand extension of away-from-home products such as paper towels, facial tissues and toilet paper that are 100% recyclable and contain a minimum of 50% post-consumer waste. This new product line was first certified with Green Seal, an NGO specializing in environmental product labels. Following this, Wausau focused its market pitch solely on the environmental message and rebranded this new product line as EcoSoft Green Seal. This marketing strategy resulted in a 44% increase in sales in the first two years in an industry that was growing at less than 3% per annum.[87]

- The management of down side risks: Measuring the environmental impact of a business allows the management to examine the supply and value chain and identify the processes and risks which have an adverse effect on resource productivity. Businesses can use this information to design eco-efficient processes that not only cut economic costs, but also have a positive environmental impact[88]. For example, IKEA, (which uses the IKEA Sustainability Scorecard - measurement framework based on the measurement of non-f inancia l performance measures) implemented a strategy for compressing items and flat-packaging. The flat packaging has allowed IKEA to optimize loads in a given truck or train, resulting in a 15% saving on fuel per item (which IKEA has passed on to customers in the form of lower prices), and a significant reduction in carbon emissions from transport.[89] Similarly, an examination of the value chain can enable businesses in identifying risks, and understand how the company affects the environment and how environmental constraints influence the company.[90]

To manage downside risks in an effective manner, businesses must improve resource productivity to get the same output with lower inputs. Furthermore, WaveRiders must cut environmental costs and regulatory burdens. Meeting regulatory requirements is expensive, both in terms of costs (for example, waste disposal, pollution control equipment, cost of fines) and resource intensity (managerial time and effort required to fill forms and ensure adherence). Finally, WaveRiders must be able to undertake eco-risk control. They must be able to identify and flag risks before they start posing a problem for the company. In order to do this, businesses must examine their supply and value chain, and see how they impact and are impacted by the environment.

One example of successful eco-risk control can be found in Nestle, which has been committed to sustainable sourcing of coffee for the last one decade. Through its Nescafe Plan released in 2010, Nestle planned to invest US$ 487 million in Sustainable Coffee Sourcing. The aim of the plan was to double the amount of beans Nestle purchased directly from farmers to 180,000 tons by 2015 and source 90,000 tons of coffee in accordance with Rainforest Alliance Principles by 2020. Moreover, the plan also stipulated that Nestle would deliver 220 million high yielding, disease-resistant plants to farmers over the next 10 years. This implied that all direct coffee purchases would meet 4C (Common Code for the Coffee Community) guidelines in 5 years.[91] Through this Nescafe Plan, Nestle also committed to establishing 300 demo farms showing best practices. Since

2010, Nestle has also provided training, equipment and support to coffee farmers.[92]

- Environmental stewardship: There are several converging trends and compelling reasons that argue for adding impact measurement to the core business strategy. Measuring and reporting environmental impact can result in the development of a strong corporate brand and reputation, which can generate customer trust and loyalty. The current business environment is characterized by new goalposts, and a complex and dynamic operating paradigm. In this environment, customer loyalty is an important consideration for creating long-term economic value. As customers pay more attention to sustainability, companies are compelled to ensure environmental compliance and make their approach visible to and inclusive of their stakeholders.

A great example of corporate environmental stewardship can be found in Walmart, which launched its Sustainability Index in 2009. Walmart uses this sustainability index to identify and reward suppliers who are using sustainable production practices. The Index comprises of 16 questions on a range of topics including greenhouse gas emissions, solid waste, water usage, community development, regulatory compliance and HR policies. Suppliers are rated on target, below target or above target depending on their responses to these questions. The company aims to use this data to rank its suppliers and slowly shift 70-80% of its business to suppliers who prioritize sustainability.[93]

This framework of upside and downside advantages presented by Esty and Winston was further validated by a set of six executive surveys conducted by McKinsey in 2011[94], which demonstrated that an increasing number of executives are acknowledging the value-creation opportunities linked to sustainability. While earlier studies found corporate reputation to be the primary driving force for embedding sustainability, the surveys revealed that achieving operational efficiency and minimizing costs (33% of executives) were the top reasons for including sustainability as a strategic driver, followed by other reasons such as reputation (32%), alignment with strategy (31%), and new growth opportunities (27%).

Similar evidence was found through an MIT Sloan Management Review and Boston Consulting Group study conducted in 2013[95]. This research is based on a survey of 1,847 executive and manager respondents from commercial enterprises. The study divides these businesses into three categories (Walkers, Talkers, On the Road) based on their responses and commitment to sustainability. Walkers focus heavily on five business fronts: sustainability strategy, business case, measurement, business model innovation and leadership commitment. Talkers, on the other hand, are equally concerned about sustainability issues, but address these issues to a lesser extent. A third group that constitutes the "On the Road" segment, is comprised of businesses that engage with some, but not all, the sustainability issues they consider significant.

The study revealed that 60% of Walker companies opined that sustainable business practices had enhanced their profitability, compared to 19% of Talker companies. The report identified that sustainability issues lay at the heart of competitive advantage and long-term viability for 'Walkers', and they considered material sustainability issues to be a "core strategic imperative".[96] The study's findings were also in line with the theory of environmental stewardship, as nearly 40% of respondents reported increased collaboration with customers and suppliers on environment and sustainability issues.

34% of respondents also said that their companies had stepped up their engagement with governments, policy makers and regulators. In some instances, businesses are even partnering with competitors to combat sustainability challenges. Examples include General Motors and Honda that are co-developing zero-emission hydrogen fuel cells to be used in each company's cars, and Ocean Spray and Tropicana who are partnering to reduce transportation costs, delivery distances, and carbon emissions.[97]

Frameworks for measuring the social, economic and environmental impact of business

Companies today have access to a variety of frameworks and tools that they can deploy to measure the socio-economic and environmental impact of their business activities. This space of measuring and reporting has matured and most of these tools are holistic in nature, as they have standards, indicators and sustainability reporting guidelines. The following overview is an illustrative one to showcase some of the more popular approaches.

1. Triple Bottom Line

When environmental sustainability started coming to the forefront in the mid 90's, John Elkington developed an accounting framework called the triple bottom line (TBL) to measure corporate performance. TBL extended beyond the traditional measures of profits, return on investment, and shareholder value to include environmental and social aspects of investment and business. Unlike traditional measures of corporate performance, TBL incorporates three dimensions of performance: social, environmental and financial. It presented a comprehensive approach for measuring corporate impact, as it assessed performance along three interrelated dimensions of people, planet, and profits.

It was a great measurement and reporting framework at the time, but the concept of TBL did not imply that it is mandatory for businesses to maximize returns across all three aspects of corporate performance. In fact, by reporting along the TBL standards, a business relays the image of sensitivity and concern for all stakeholders, but clearly maintains that businesses cannot be successful if they disregard the interests of external and internal stakeholders. The fundamental premise was a long-term sustainability one. Put simply, in order to be successful in the long run, businesses have to sustain profitability over all three dimensions which requires that the whole impact of the company's commercial activities must be measured, reported and assessed on a regular basis. It followed a model similar to the financial reporting model and schedule that most companies adhere to, making it easier to understand and adopt for most.

Owing to the diverse nature of the dimensions included in the TBL approach, there are no universally accepted standard measures for calculating each TBL dimension. Nevertheless, performance under each dimension was broadly defined as demonstrated in the table below.

Performance Areas under Triple Bottom Line Approach

Economic Performance	This can be divided into operational and financial performance. Operational performance includes variables such as market share, product quality, and marketing effectiveness. On the other hand, financial performance encompasses market-based performance (e.g., stock price, dividend payout and earnings per share) and accounting-based performance (e.g., return on assets and return on equity).[98]
Environmental Performance	This dimension of corporate performance refers to the amount of resources (e.g. energy, land, water) a business uses in its operations, and the impact its activities have on the environment (e.g. emissions, water wastage, chemical residue).
Social Performance	This refers to the impact of a business on the community in which it operates. This includes dimensions such as jobs created, working conditions, employee satisfaction, and so on.

Source: Triple Bottom Line" as "Sustainable Corporate Performance": A Proposition for the Future. Hasan Fauzi, Goran Svensson, and Azhar Abdul Rahman. Sustainability, 2(5), 1345-1360. 2010.

As cor porations of all sizes become increasingly socially and environmentally conscious, many of these businesses are pursuing the triple bottom line. One example is DHL, which is now using couriers on bicycles in Germany and the Netherlands to reduce carbon dioxide emissions. Some companies are even going a step ahead by volunteering to be held accountable to the triple bottom line and becoming benefit corporations that include social and environmental performance as legally defined goals. Patagonia, an outdoor apparel and accessory firm, became a benefit organization in 2012. The company does not use any chemicals in their production processes and often use recycled, organic, or environmentally friendly materials.[99]

2. OECD Guidelines for Multinational Enterprises (MNE Guidelines)

The OECD MNE Guidelines are one of the most comprehensive international frameworks for ensuring that businesses adhere to responsible conduct. The Guidelines represent an international reference document that contains recommendations from governments to their MNEs on responsible business conduct at home and abroad. A unique feature of the Guidelines is an implementation mechanism which is based on National Contact Points (NCPs) established by adhering governments. The NCP's mandate is to promote the MNE Guidelines, and offer a non-judicial grievance mechanism that can resolve issues that arise as the Guidelines are implemented. The Guidelines include voluntary standards and principles that cover a range of areas including human rights, employment and labour issues, disclosure of information, anti-corruption, and taxation compliance. In the sustainability context, it gives specific focus to two topics, environment and disclosure of information.

- Environment: This section provides recommendations for MNEs to continuously improve their environmental performance and take due account of the need to protect the environment, public health and safety, and generally to conduct their activities in a manner contributing to the wider goal of sustainable development. They also urge enterprises to maximize their contribution to environmental protection by undertaking environmental risk management.
- Disclosure of Information: This chapter recommends that enterprises ensure that timely and accurate information is disclosed on all material matters regarding their activities, structure, financial situation, performance, ownership and governance. This information should be disclosed for the enterprise as a whole, and, where appropriate, along business lines or geographic areas.

The OECD MNE Guidelines are a comprehensive instrument for responsible business conduct. They are all-inclusive in nature, and are not restricted to large corporations only. They can also be applied to small and medium-sized businesses that are active in more than one country[100]. The Guidelines also recommend that MNEs should seek to avoid adverse impacts of their own business activities in the areas covered by the Guidelines. Avoiding adverse impact can be achieved on many fronts ranging from[101] not being the direct cause of an adverse impact, to encouraging business partners (along the supply chain) to adopt responsible corporate behavior.

The global reach and adherence to OECD Guidelines has increased significantly since their introduction in 1976. Currently, 35 OECD and 11 non-OECD countries adhere to the Guidelines. As of 2016, 44 out of the 46 countries had established NCPs, which were actively involved in undertaking promotional activities, handling enquiries and contributing to the resolution of issues related to the Guidelines in specific instances. Stakeholders such as NGOs, trade unions, and local community organizations can use the NCP system to submit their grievances and/or specific instances against companies that do not adhere to the Guidelines. NCPs examine the case and take action against companies, often asking them to resolve the dispute at hand, consider the grievance, and re-examine their impacts and CSR strategies in light of the grievance.

NCP System in Practice: The Case of Michelin Group

> In July 2012, the French NCP received a request for review from four NGOs and a trade union alleging that Michelin Group, a French multinational enterprise, did not adhere to the general policies, disclosure, human rights, employment and industrial relations, environment, and combating bribery provisions of the OECD MNE Guidelines in India. They highlighted that the company had constructed a tire manufacturing plant on recently industrialized pasture land, which was having negative effects on local populations.

> The French NCP undertook a detailed analysis of the company's behavior in relation to the Guidelines. The NCP concluded that the Michelin Group did not violate the OECD Guidelines, although several recommendations of the OECD Guidelines were not adequately complied with or not fully implemented. As a consequence of the consultation with the company and the parties reporting the grievance, the Michelin Group undertook preparatory steps for environmental, social and human rights impact assessment studies for the industrial project in Tamil Nadu (India). The Michelin Group also committed to developing an action plan to adapt its CSR policy and internal due diligence systems in response to the outcomes of the studies.

Source: *Michelin Group, and four NGOs and a trade union. OECD. 2016*

3. Global Reporting Initiative (GRI) Reporting Framework

The GRI Reporting Framework aims to serve as a generally accepted framework that an organization can use to report its economic/financial, environmental, and social performance.[102] It is designed to be applicable for businesses of all sizes and across sectors and locations. It comprises of general and sector-specific standards and principles that have been developed after consulting with a wide range of stakeholders. The Framework also contains Sustainability Reporting Guidelines, which define the content and quality of the report's content.[103] Standard disclosures made up of performance indicators (covering criteria on energy, biodiversity and emissions) are also included in the framework.

Moreover, the Framework also contains indicator protocols (i.e. definitions, compilation guidance, other information to ensure consistency), sector supplements (i.e. guidance on how to apply the Guidelines in a specific sector), and technical protocols (i.e. reporting process)[104].

GRI Reporting Framework

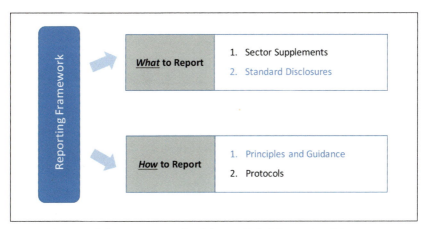

Source: Sustainability Reporting Guidelines. Global Reporting Initiative.

The indicators within the GRI Guidelines range from the organizational vision and profile of companies to their sustainability governance and protocols for identifying and addressing unethical behavior or other matters of integrity. The indicators are divided into three main categories, namely economic, environmental, and social. Social impact is sub-divided into four categories - labor practices and decent work, human rights, society, and product responsibility.

Performance Areas	Performance Indicators/Aspects of Performance
1. Economic	• Economic performance (economic value generated and distributed) • Market presence (e.g. spending on locally-based suppliers) • Indirect economic impacts (e.g. investments made for public benefit)

Performance Areas	Performance Indicators/Aspects of Performance
2. Environment	- Materials (amount of new and recycled material) - Energy (efficiency, conservation, usage) - Water (amount of water withdrawn, recycled and re-used) - Biodiversity (use of areas of high biodiversity value, strategy for managing impact on biodiversity) - Emissions, effluents, and waste - Products and services - Compliance (value of fines imposed for non-compliance) - Transport (impact on environment) - Environmental protection expenditures & investments
3. Social	
3A. Labor Practices and Decent Work	- Employment (total employment generated, benefits) - Labor/management relations - Occupational health and safety - Training and education - Diversity and equal opportunity - Equal remuneration for women and men
3B. Human Rights	- Investment and procurement practices - Non-discrimination - Freedom of association and collective bargaining - Child labor - Forced and compulsory labor - Security practices - Indigenous rights - Assessment - Remediation

Performance Areas	Performance Indicators/Aspects of Performance
3C. Society	• Local communities (impact, mitigation measures) • Corruption • Public policy (participation in policy development, financial and in-kind contributions to political actors and institutions) • Anti-competitive behavior • Compliance
3D. Product Responsibility	• Customer health and safety • Product and service labelling • Marketing communications • Customer privacy • Compliance

Source: *Sustainability Reporting Guidelines. Global Reporting Initiative. 2011.*

While this list of indicators is exhaustive, it is recognized that the capacity of different companies to report will vary, depending on how long they have been reporting for. To address this, GRI Guidelines allow companies to report to different levels - each level reflecting a different level of use of the GRI Framework. Companies who are new to reporting can report at Level C, and produce a report comprising of ten material indicators (including at least one indicator from economic, environmental and social). These companies can start as beginners (Level C) and move to higher levels with time.[105] Companies are also encouraged not to report in silos but to focus on the value chain, and report the impact they have through these value chains[106]. However, companies that are relatively new to reporting can determine the boundaries of their reports, often to material issues impacted by the company's own facilities only. On the other hand, bigger companies like Nestle prepare a comprehensive report with 17 indicators, in accordance with the GRI's G4 guidelines.

The Guidelines comprise of Reporting Principles, Reporting Guidance, and Standard Disclosures (including Performance Indicators). The Reporting Principles describe the outcomes a report should achieve and guide decisions throughout the reporting process (e.g. selecting which topics and Indicators to report on and how to report on them).

There are two groups of principles, both of which are in place to help ensure transparency in sustainability reporting:

GRI's Reporting Principles	
Principles for identifying the topics and indicators for reporting	**Materiality:** The report should include information that reflects the organization's economic, environmental, and social impacts, and would influence the assessments and decisions of stakeholders significantly.
	Stakeholder inclusiveness: The reporting company should identify key stakeholders and ex plain i n the report how it has responded to their reasonable expectations and interests.
	Sustainability context: The report should present the organization's performance in the wider context of sustainability.
	Completeness: The company should define the report boundary and cover all the relevant indicators to ensure that all the significant economic, environmental, and social impacts are covered.
Principles for quality assurance and presentation of the reported information	**Comparability:** Issues and information should be selected, compiled, and reported consistently.
	Accuracy: The reported information should be sufficiently accurate and detailed for stakeholders to assess the reporting organization's performance.
	Timeliness: Reporting is undertaken consistently and according to a schedule. The information is available in time for stakeholders to make informed decisions.
	Clarity: Stakeholders should be able to access and understand the information presented in the report.
	Reliability: The methodology and information used to prepare the report should be gathered, recorded, compiled, analyzed, and disclosed in a way that could be subject to examination and that establishes the quality and materiality of the information.

Once the business has identified the appropriate scope and indicators of the report, it must determine which entities' (e.g., subsidiaries and joint ventures) performance will be represented by the report. The Sustainability Report Boundary should clearly specify the entities over which the business has control or significant influence via upstream and downstream entities.

In terms of global coverage, at present, GRI is the most widely adopted framework for corporate reporting. 63% of N100 companies and 75% of G250 companies are using the GRI framework to report their performance. The number of businesses that have already adopted the GRI Standards is also on the rise. Currently, 111 policies across 50 countries and regions reference GRI, and 89 training partners across 54 countries offer GRI Certified Training Courses. A total of 30,525 practitioners have been trained to use the GRI reporting framework to date – up from a mere 358 in 2008. The majority of these practitioners are from the Americas (14,314), followed by Asia and Oceania (7,789), Europe (6,965) and Africa (1,457).[107]

4. Integrated Reporting

The first company to adopt an integrated reporting approach was the Danish biotechnology company Novozymes. Produced in 2002, Novozymes' first integrated report provided information about areas that the company considered important for the majority of its stakeholders. The report declared that moving forward, Novozymes would focus on reporting along three bottom lines namely financial, environmental, and social impact of its corporate activities. The decision to embed all three impact areas in one report was made in the wake of increased interaction between sustainability and business, and was driven by the stakeholders' demand for a wider overview of the business. While many argue that this pioneering effort was a combined rather than integrated report, it is safe to conclude that it was a progressive step to entrench sustainability as a key performance indicator. The report disclosed Novozymes' performance in non-financial areas (social, environmental and knowledge development/innovation indicators), and the company's consideration of non-investor stakeholders showed that it was laying the groundwork for a truly integrated report.[108]

Another company that has been producing integrated reports for over a decade is Royal Philips Electronics - a company that works in multiple sectors including healthcare, lighting and lifestyle. In 2008, Philips introduced integrated reporting for its annual report and embedding sustainability as a key driver for its growth. The primary impetus behind this integrated reporting approach was to ensure transparency and present a unified and holistic picture of the company's performance. Quantitative and qualitative aspects of the sustainability issues were embedded in the report, which showcased various ESG (environmental, social and governance) metrics including measures of customer satisfaction and loyalty, employee engagement, sales of green products and the company's carbon footprint. Moving forward, starting in 2009, the report included economic indicators in sustainability performance, sustainability risks and opportunities, and the amount invested by Philips in green innovations.[109]

In the US, Southwest Airlines is one of the first companies that started issuing an integrated report. Since 2010, Southwest has been producing a yearly integrated report that follows a triple bottom line structure, focusing on performance, people, and planet. Their report includes a two-page summary table summarizing the multiple indicators used to measure the company's track record in each area. Southwest's One Report also presents stories illustrating key strategic efforts and indicators in each area. The different types of capitals covered in the report include fixed and financial capital, as well as digital, human, relationship, and natural capitals. The performance section includes coverage of full financials, focusing particularly on ROIC as the main metric. Detailed information about airplane fleet and management is also included in this section. In the people's section, the report covers Southwest's various stakeholders including employees, customers, community, and suppliers. The planet section includes the company's environmental impacts such as energy, fuel and water consumption, regulatory complia nce, conservation, waste management and recycling.[110]

While the uptake of integrated reporting is low in Asia, there has nevertheless been significant progress in the last few years. In 2015,

City Developments Limited (CDL) became the first property developer in Singapore to adopt this approach. Their approach is centered around six types of capital, including financial, manufactured, organizational, social and relationship, human and natural capital. Its integrated reporting approach replaced the traditional annual report that focused exclusively on financial and stock market performance of the company. With this new approach, CDL aimed to start presenting a more holistic picture of the company's performance to its stakeholders and investors, and describe the relationship between the company's business and sustainability performance, and how this generates value in the short and long term. The specific financial, social, and environmental issues covered in the integrated report have been determined through an assessment conducted with internal and external stakeholders including customers, business associates, employees, builders and suppliers, as well as government organizations. With regard to environmental performance, CDL has included metrics such as reduction in carbon emissions and water usage, increase in renewable energy generated by CDL-managed buildings, and the total savings in electricity bills.[111]

5. WBCSD Measuring Impact Framework

World Business Council for Sustainable Development (WBCSD)[112] is a global organization led by CEOs of over 200 leading global businesses working together to catalyze the transition to a sustainable world. Member companies are from different economic sectors and all major economies, and span across the value chain. Some prominent member companies include Acer, Bloomberg, BMW Group, Dupont, Roche, Ikea, Shell, Novartis, Unilever and Apple Inc. The common goal is to create high-impact solutions to sustainability challenges in their respective areas of operation.

In 2006, upon the request of member companies, the WBCSD started developing a framework to assess the economic and development impact of business in the societies where it operates. It was designed to assist companies in understanding their contribution to development, and utilize this information to guide decision-making and engage with stakeholders in a more informed manner. While the framework does not offer a corporate reporting mechanism, it can be used to improve the quality of reporting and communication with external audiences and stakeholders[113].

This framework was a departure from previous frameworks in the sense that it was done with a business-first lens. It is grounded in what business does, as has been developed by business for business. More importantly, it extends beyond compliance, and emphasizes what positive contributions businesses can have beyond traditional reporting. The Framework encourages stakeholder engagement and open dialogue with the objective of creating a shared perspective of business impacts and societal needs. It also aims to understand the capacity of businesses to address these needs.

It is also characterized by being (a) flexible in that it can be adapted by any business from any industry/country at any stage of the business cycle, and (b) complementary in that it complements existing measurement tools, frameworks and standards (e.g. GRI Reporting Initiative and IFC Performance Standards).

The methodology of the Framework integrates the economic and social contributions of a business's activities and operations[114]. Business activities are categorized into four clusters, namely (i) governance and sustainability; (ii) assets, (iii) people; and (iv) financial flows.

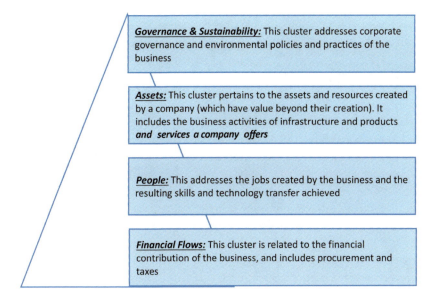

The Framework is based on a four-step methodology[115]:

1. Set Boundaries: The company determines the objectives, scope and depth of the assessment, answering questions related to geographical boundary and types of business activities to be addressed.
2. Measure Direct and Indirect Impacts: As a second step, the company identifies and measures its footprint (direct and indirect impacts), and also explores what the company can control and influence through its business activities.
3. Assess Contribution to Development: In this step, the company examines the (direct and indirect) development impacts of its business and operations. The Framework also encourages the company to engage with stakeholders to prioritize development issues and build the hypothesis of the business's contribution to development in the area of operation.
4. Prioritize Management Response: The company conducts an analysis of risks and opportunities and identifies priority areas for action. Possible management responses are considered and strategies are developed. Moreover, the way forward is decided and the company formulates performance indicators to monitor progress.

> Applying the WBCSD Measuring Impact Framework – The Case of Eskom, South Africa
>
> Eskom is a state-owned utility operating in South Africa. It is a vertically integrated body that is the country's largest electricity producer, generating approximately 95% of electricity used in South Africa and approximately 45% of electricity used across the continent. Eskom's aim is to provide electricity solutions in an efficient and sustainable manner. In an effort to measure its footprint in South Africa, Eskom started a comprehensive assessment of the economic, social and environmental impact, both positive and negative, of its activities. The assessment is based on the WBCSD Measuring Impact Framework, which was applied within the Eskom's specific context. Eskom used the 4-step process to define its economic, social and environmental impact along the three key stages of the utility's major activities, namely (i) the construction of new power plants, (ii) the generation, transmission, distribution and retailing of electricity, and (iii) the usage of electricity by customers.
>
> As a first step, Eskom applied the Framework to identify its South African operations as the main boundary of the assessment. The second step involved identifying and measuring, where possible, the direct and indirect impacts arising from the company's activities and mapping out what impacts are within the control of the company and what it can influence through its business. An impact tree was used to facilitate the identification of impacts. To illustrate, an activity generates the first level of impact. These key sources or drivers of impact – for instance the use of resources – further branch out into more specific areas of indirect impacts, i.e. water usage, use of land. At the next level, the methodology includes concrete measurable indicators for each impact. In this example, liters of water used and square meters of the different types of land employed are quantified. Based on these numbers, it is possible to then judge whether the overall impact is positive or negative. The same process is followed for each first-level impact. Through this process, more than 150 indicators were identified, evaluated and consolidated to determine Eskom's overall footprint. Following this, six key areas of influence where Eskom's economic, social and environmental footprint helps to shape South Africa's development were identified.

Source: Measuring Eskom's footprint in South Africa. WBCSD. http://wbcsdpublications.org/wp-content/uploads/2016/02/WBCSD-case-study-Eskom-Factor.pdf. 2016

The Age of Sustainability: From Millennium to Sustainable Development Goals

Companies around the world are moving to measuring and reporting their impact from various lenses. Irrespective of motivation, what is obvious is that they recognize that financial data alone cannot satisfy the stakeholders' need for information. Companies are adopting a more holistic view to measure and report the socio-economic and environmental contributions of their business activities[116]. This is indeed the rising age of sustainability.

At a global level, and led by the United Nations, the transition from Millennium Development Goals (MDGs) to Sustainable Development Goals (SDGs) provided greater thrust to this trend for measuring and reporting impact. Unlike the MDGs, the SDGs explicitly called on businesses to mobilize and apply their wealth, creativity and innovation to develop solutions to make development sustainable. As the engine of economic growth and employment, business can accelerate progress towards sustainable development[117]. From the business perspective, SDGs present an opportunity for companies to develop and implement solutions and technologies that solve sustainability challenges facing the world today. They encourage companies to develop a competitive advantage for themselves by exhibiting how their business activities forward the sustainable development agenda by reducing negative impacts and maximizing positive impact. In doing this, the SDGs "connect business strategies with global priorities" for sustainable development[118]. By using the SDGs as a central framework to formulate, implement and communicate their strategies, companies can gain on many fronts[119]. They can identify future business opportunities as the SDGs redirect global public and private investment flows towards key sustainability challenges. They will also incentivize innovation by encouraging companies to use resources more efficiently and transition to more sustainable alternatives. Supporting the SDGs will also definitely strengthen stakeholder relations. The SDGs are a composite representation of stakeholder expectations and the policy direction that will be taken at regional, national and international levels. As such, they present an opportunity for companies to align their growth priorities and business strategies with future policies and stakeholder needs.

Moreover, SDGs have the potential to stabilize markets. For businesses to succeed, it is important that the societies in which they operate have rules-based markets, transparent financial systems, and well-governed institutions. The national and international commitment to invest in the SDGs is likely to strengthen these basic pillars for business success, thus benefiting companies in the longer term[120]. Hence, businesses are seen as both the drivers and beneficiaries of sustainable development.

Within sustainable development, the environment is a key area of focus, both for businesses and for governments. While the MDGs achieved great success in reducing poverty and hunger, improving social outcomes in education and health[121], and improving overall material wellbeing of millions around the world, the MDGs had limited coverage of environment sustainability issues. The one goal (MDG-7) that focused on the environment only considered reducing the consumption of ozone depleting substances, and improving access to drinking water and sanitation. Problems pertaining to air and water pollution, accumulation of chemical wastes, and the continual unsustainable use of natural resources were not addressed. While slowing down the loss of biodiversity was included as a target, progress towards achievement of this was limited. Overall, studies show that the formulation of MDG-7 was weak, and that weakness translated into uneven and scarce implementation[122].

In fact, progress in achieving other MDGs had unintended negative consequences for the environment. For example, reducing poverty and hunger were in many cases, achieved through modern agriculture, which required significantly more water, and was reliant on synthetic chemical fertilizers and use of machinery. Crop cultivation practices resulted in pesticide contamination of neighboring ecosystems, an increase in the emission of greenhouse gases, as well as other air pollutants, and eutrophication of surface waters and coastal zones.

Deforestation was also undertaken to expand cropland to provide more food[123].

Thus, while the economic and social targets of the MDGs were met to a great extent, this development came at the expense of less focus on environmental sustainability. Furthermore, as the balance of natural eco-systems deteriorated, climate-change caused significantly more natural catastrophes in the decade leading up to 2015. In 2014 alone, half of the 28 weather extremes (including floods, snowstorms, and heatwaves) recorded around the world were attributed to human-induced climate change[124]. In the wake of these challenges, the SDGs were designed to emphasize environmental sustainability as a key development objective.

As the SDGs were launched, governments around the world started using them as a roadmap to reshape their national policy and implement regulations supporting the achievement of the goals. The Government of Finland, for example, set up a multi-stakeholder SDG Commission led by the Finnish Prime Minister. Other countries like the United Arab Emirates restructured the Ministry of Environment into a Ministry of Environment and Climate Change.

A notable example at the national level was undertaken in Germany, where a Council for Sustainable Development was established to advise the Federal Government on sustainable development[125]. Operating as an independent council, it advises the government on its sustainable development policy and, by presenting proposals for targets and indicators, seeks to advance the Sustainability Strategy as well as propose projects for its realization. The Council also fosters social dialogue on the issue of sustainability to increase the level of awareness among all concerned and the population as to what sustainable development actually means by demonstrating the consequences of social action and discussing possible solutions.

The Council's current work programme[126] includes various areas like digitalization and the opportunities it creates for sustainable development in our society, the funding of sustainable development (Green Finance), sustainable towns and cities, and strategies for practical action on sustainability. The Council also deals with governance, i.e. the political steer for the implementation of the Government's Sustainable Development Strategy. Agenda 2030 with its Sustainable Development Goals (SDGs) and the German Sustainability Strategy provide the framework for the Council's activities.

It is clear from these examples that sustainability is becoming core to national strategies around the world, and the trend continues to expand as governments like Australia and Canada publish reports analyzing the opportunities and challenges that arise as a result of employing the SDG framework in their national policies[127].

Sustainability and business: a win-win relation

Faced with volatile supply chains and other challenges rooted in climate change, many global businesses realized that making a profit while simultaneously benefiting society had the potential to generate viable and scalable solutions. In addition, business leaders understood that embedding sustainability in their core strategies could also improve bottom line results in the long term and create greater value for investors and shareholders.

One, simple, and good example in this context is PepsiCo's innovation in energy consumption[128]. PepsiCo owns one of the largest fleets of all electric delivery trucks. In 2014, they managed to save over US$ 3 million while also reducing emissions by more than 20% as compared to conventional diesel engines.

Embracing this potential of environmentally sound policies, business models and range of products and services marked a great shift in the perception of business viz-a-vis sustainability. Companies that had historically viewed sustainability as a side issue started aligning their business strategies with the SDGs to maintain a competitive advantage over other companies that had not realized the economic potential of sustainable solutions. Smart companies also realized that the policy and regulatory environment they operate in will, sooner or later, be affected by the SDGs. This, in turn, will fundamentally alter the operating environment for business and companies that accept those facts and embrace it early will have an advantage[129].

Integrating sustainability into existing industrial facilities is a tall task. Ford built its River Rouge plant in 1917, and made the decision to upgrade it and make it more sustainable in the year 2000. In addition to a modernization exercise, Ford invested in a "living roof"[130]. 90% of the truck plant final assembly building was covered with plants, mainly drought-resistant species of sedum. Ford's leadership considered this decision to be one driven by financial and economic gains rather than a corporate sustainability initiative. Underlying the decision to set up this living roof was an innovative water management plan. The landscape-based infrastructure would cost Ford less as it involves minimum usage of pipes. Moreover, the roof would serve as a natural filter of rainwater, thus reducing the need for chemical-based treatment. Excess storm water could also be managed effectively through this infrastructure, as the vegetation had the ability to absorb one inch of water. The green roof was also expected to act as a natural temperature controller, as it would keep the building at least 10 degrees cooler in the summer months and 10 degrees warmer in the winter – thus resulting in a 5% reduction in energy costs for the plant. Plants would also produce oxygen which could offset the company's carbon emissions. Furthermore, the roof required less maintenance compared to a standard roof, and would provide a thriving natural habitat for birds, butterflies and insects, therefore maintaining biodiversity in the vicinity.

Evidence on global business performance also shows that companies that place emphasis on environmental, social and governance factors, and are trying to integrate sustainable business practices stand to gain, both in the short and the long term. Short term advantages include lower costs of debt and equity, as the market recognizes them as low risk and rewards them accordingly. According to research findings, companies that integrate sustainability into risk mitigation and improved communication and collaboration with their stakeholders attract more funding than their less responsible counterparts.[131]

In the medium to long term, these companies typically outperform the market in terms of net returns and corporate financial performance. Companies report that sustainability strategies also generate value by decreasing operational and regulatory risk, as well as reducing operation and supply chain costs. Moreover, businesses stand to gain a greater market share or price premiums, and growth via new markets or product innovation by integrating sustainability in their business planning and practices. It challenges businesses to think beyond profit and be more creative to solve a new set of problems and generate innovation.[132] In fact, a survey of 250 CFOs conducted in 2012 found that 32% of senior executives expect more than 5% of future annual revenue growth to come from products and services that reduce environmental and social impacts.[133]

The example of Danone is a compelling one in terms of how sustainability drove the development of a new product and uncovered a new stream of revenue for a company. In 2005, Danone and Grameen Bank created Grameen Danone Foods Ltd (GDFL), with the aim of establishing a small yoghurt plant in Bogra, Bangladesh. The plant would promote local development and bring health to the community. The main product manufactured by the plant was a yoghurt which is fortified with zinc, iron, iodine, vitamin A, and accounts for 30% of a child's recommended daily nutrients. The milk for producing the yogurt comes from local micro-farmers; and the yoghurts are distributed by a network of Rural Sales Women, commonly known as Jita. In addition to the health benefits it was to bring to the community, the plant also generated employment for plant workers, women distributors and the farmers supplying the milk for the yogurt. For Danone, the project offered an opportunity to innovate and develop a low-cost nutritious product, widen its range of consumers, and learn new marketing techniques to sell a product to a completely new market segment, i.e. low-income households in Bangladesh.[134]

Companies around the world are seeking to be Net Positive and give back to society and the environment. To counter the rapid rate of resource extraction, real estate and construction companies are now embracing sustainability with new vigor. With more and more buildings coming up around the world each year, the real estate and construction sector's eco-footprint has a large impact on the natural world. While carbon-neutrality has been featuring on the strategies of many companies in the sector for some time now, some companies in the sector are going an extra mile and adopting a Net Positive approach to put back more into society and the planet than they take out. They are focusing on opportunities that can provide solutions to environmental and socio- economic problems while also generating a profit, thus making perfect business sense.

Global sector leaders such as Lendlease, Mirvac, Berkeley Group, and most recently Hammerson, have made Net Positive commitments. These commitments vary in terms of their scope and the depth of issues covered. While some are concentrating on landlord-controlled activities or development-specific impacts, others are extending the frontier and undertaking sustainable reform up and down their value chains[135]. These companies strive to be Net Positive in particular areas, such as carbon emissions or water usage. However, some companies are setting bigger goals. In London, Lendlease is working in partnership with Southwark Council to deliver a regeneration programme on 28 acres of land in the centre of Elephant & Castle.[136] Situated in London's Zone 1, the project's vision is to create Central London's new green heart. In addition to a design that supports carbon efficiency, Lendlease has designed a zero-carbon heat and power system for the entire community and invested in behavioural change campaigns to further bring down energy and water use.[137]

Hammerson has also launched its business-wide commitment to achieve Net Positive across a range of issues, including carbon and resource use, by 2030. This commitment will see it take on the major challenge of tackling its equity share of impacts over which it has direct control, as well as those of its tenants and major joint venture investments – Value Retail and VIA Outlets.[138] To achieve this, the company will be splitting this goal out into five-year budgets or milestones, beginning with landlord-controlled activities. Simultaneously, Hammerson will also be setting up a programme of strategic partnerships with key stakeholders, such as tenants, to significantly reduce their impacts – a process made easier by the knowledge that 10 tenants alone represent nearly half of all tenant electricity emissions.[139]

Businesses around the world have indeed come along way, from looking at environmental issues as a distraction or public relations exercise, to adopting a full sustainable strategy (not only environmental, but overall sustainability). A sustainable strategy for a company is one that enables it to create value for shareholders over the long term while contributing to a sustainable society. In doing so, it must balance the needs of different types of providers of financial capital (e.g., shareholders and debt holders) and stakeholders representing various environmental and social interests of civil society. Typically tradeoffs are involved, although these can be reduced or even reversed through innovation.

The Real Estate Sector: Going Green

As the role and profile of sustainability increased across sectors, governments around the world started focusing on the real estate and construction sector. The sector accounts for 5-10% of the national GDP of each country in the world. Furthermore, as assets, buildings represent 50% of global wealth. It is also a sector with a considerable and increasing environmental footprint. Currently, the real estate and construction sector uses more energy than any other sector and according to most estimates, it is one of the leading contributors of carbon emissions. 20% of all greenhouse gas emissions originate from buildings, and by 2030, carbon emissions from buildings are projected to increase by 56%.

Types of Building Greenhouse Gases (GHG) Emissions[140]

Type of Emissions	Description
Direct emission sources from buildings	These are emissions from all the GHG sources located physically in the building, mainly fossil-fuel consuming equipment (e.g. boilers, oil lamps...), as well as heating and cooling systems using Fluorinated F-Gas, and marginally, from insulation material. Cooking with gas or fuel also accounts as a major source of GHG emissions.
Indirect emissions sources from building energy consumption	Mainly building electricity use, plus commercial heat from district heating and cooling. The electrical demand in buildings induces GHG emissions in the power sector. Electrical uses include notably: the consumption by electrical equipment that are incorporated in the building (e.g. heating and cooling systems, electric lighting, elevators, pumps) and consumption of electrical goods (e.g. household appliances) and other related service equipment (e.g. IT goods).
Buildings' indirect emissions from other sources	Mainly concerns embedded emissions from building materials and the GHG emissions generated by urban planning decisions (e.g. unnecessary travel or traffic induced by building location).

In addition to these emissions, the sector annually consumes over 40% of global energy, and 40% of raw materials globally (amounting to 3 billion tonnes). These raw materials are extracted, processed, transported, added in the construction phase, and disposed. Thus, there are environmental implications at every stage of the construction life cycle. In terms of freshwater usage, by 2030, buildings are expected to use 12% of global freshwater, and generate circa 30% of total waste[141].

Projecting forward, the real estate sector is poised for continuing growth. Global demographic and socio-economic forces such as the rapid increase in population and urbanization are likely to drive this growth. Today, more than half of the world's population now lives in towns and cities, and by 2030, 60% (approximately 4.9 billion people) will live in urban environments. The largest cities, which are expected to contribute 61% of global GDP will need 260 million new homes, and 540 million square meters of new office space. The rising purchasing power in emerging economies will further stimulate demand for buildings and consequently increase the demand for energy by 50% by 2050[142]. In response to this demand, global construction output is expected to reach US$ 15.5 trillion (3.9% CAGR) by 2030[143]. If nothing changes, this will cause a major challenge to global emissions, waste, and sustainability (or lack of in this case).

Moreover, it is imperative to note that climate change will also affect existing buildings. Natural weather-related hazards such as storms, flooding and seepages will compromise the durability of some building materials and magnify the risk of collapse or damage. This, in turn, will reduce building lifetime, while simultaneously increasing the incidence of health-related issues caused by worsening indoor climate[144].

Keeping in view the environmental footprint of the industry, green standards and principles were developed by international organizat ions and governments to ensure that the industry's practices were environmentally sustainable. Meanwhile, the real estate and construction sector has also acknowledged the importance of environmental sustainability in its decision-making. Companies in the sector are increasingly inclined towards green buildings and environmentally sustainable construction and operational practices. According to estimates, 40-48% of new commercial builds in 2016 were "green", showing a marked increase from a mere 2% in 2005. As specifications and related regulations are more strictly enforced, this percentage is expected to increase to 55% in 2020. While it is difficult to make the existing stock of buildings more environmentally sustainable, retrofitting efforts have nevertheless been undertaken by the industry to produce greener properties. It is expected that by 2020, 13% of total carbon emissions savings will be generated by retrofitted buildings. In terms of energy usage, as one example, 46% of commercial buildings will be covered by LED lighting by 2020[145].

This movement led to the rise of sustainable property developers who proved the viable economics of going green. Singapore-listed CDL is a global leader in sustainability[146]. Since adopting its ethos of "Conserving as we Construct" in 1995, the property development and investment company has become an industry pioneer in green building innovation - creating the first eco-mall and condominium in Singapore, and first CarbonNeutral development in Asia Pacific. Its developments prioritize energy efficiency, including the deployment of the largest solar panel in a Singapore condominium block. Leveraging its position as one of Singapore's biggest landlords, CDL's sustainability efforts do not cease at the construction phase. The company regularly engages its tenants, homebuyers, youths and the community in the adoption of environmentally responsible practices.

As was the case with all other industries, the uptake of green practices in the real estate and construction industry was driven by a combination of stakeholder demand and business gains, namely lower operating costs and improvement in brand reputation. Regulation, of course, is one of the main driving factors. Surveys conducted by the World Green Building Council show a strong correlation between the prevalence and coverage of national regulation and the percentage of green building activity in each country[147].

Triggers driving future green buildings activity % - 2008/2012

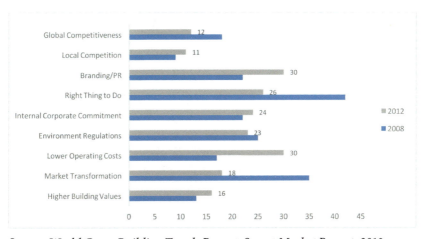

Source: World Green Building Trends Report, Smart Market Report, 2013

Sustainability reporting in the real estate and construction industry has also improved alongside the uptake of sustainable building practices. The Global Real Estate Sustainability Benchmark (GRESB), which is the global standard for assessing sustainability in the real estate, conducts annual surveys to analyze the sustainability performance of 707 companies in the real estate and construction sector. The 2015

GRESB Survey shows that 348 out of 707 property companies and funds have long-term energy reduction targets, and 10 companies and funds have reduction targets of 50% (or more), over an average period of 11 years[148], among many other encouraging plans and targets for improving their environmental footprint.

While there are differences between sub-sectors in the extent to which sustainability is embedded into business practices and operations, the consistent improvement in sustainability performance and reporting cannot be denied. However, given that the sector is one of the most significant contributors to carbon emissions, energy consumption and raw material consumption, more concrete measures are needed.

(Endnotes)

63 The Davos 2018 environment agenda - what you need to know and how to follow online. https://www.weforum.org/agenda/2018/01/the-davos-2018-environment-agenda-online-what-you-need-to-know/. January 2018

64 Time for west to adjust to 'new normal'. Andrew Sentence. Financial Times. June 30, 2012. https://www.ft.com/content/9213d8a4-d4d4-11e1-b476-00144feabdc0

65 2017 Hurricane Season Was the Most Expensive in U.S. History. National Geographic. https://news.nationalgeographic.com/2017/11/2017-hurricane-season-most-expensive-us-history-spd/. November 2017.

66 The Davos 2018 environment agenda - what you need to know and how to follow online. https://www.weforum.org/agenda/2018/01/the-davos-2018-environment-agenda-online-what-you-need-to-know/. January 2018

67 Germany Makes Climate Action a Key Focus of G20 Presidency Main Points, Agenda and Initiatives. United Nations Framework Convention on Climate Change. http://newsroom.unfccc.int/unfccc-newsroom/germany-makes-climate-action-key-focus-of-g20-presidency/. 2017.

68 8 in 10 people now see climate change as a 'catastrophic risk': survey. https://HYPERLINK http://www.reuters.com/article/us-climatechange-risk- www.reuters.com/article/us-climatechange-risk- survey/8-in-10-people-now-see-climate-change-as-a-catastrophic-risk-survey-idUSKBN18J36O. May 2017

69 Global Catastrophic Risks. Global Challenges Foundation. 2016

70 Reducing Pollution. The World Bank. HYPERLINK http://www.worldbank.org/ http://www.worldbank.org/en/topic/environment/brief/pollution. April 2017

71 Green Generation: Millenials Say Sustainability is a Shopping Priority. HYPERLINK http://w/ http://www.nielsen.com/pk/en/insights/news/2015/green-generation-millennials-say-sustainability-is-a-shopping-priority.html. 2015.

72 Millennials Going Green Means Retail Must Follow. Total Retail. HYPERLINK http://w/ http://www.mytotalretail.com/article/millennials-going-green-means-retail-must-follow/. May 2017

73 Millennials Going Green Means Retail Must Follow. Total Retail. HYPERLINK http://w/ http://w w w.my totalretail.com/article/millennials-going-gree n-means-retail-must-follow/. May 2017
74 Measuring and managing total impact: A new language for business decisions. PwC. 2013.
75 Green to gold: how smart companies use environmental strategy to innovate, create value, and build competitive advantage. Daniel Esty and Andrew Winston. Hoboken, NJ: John Wiley & Sons. 2009.
76 GE's Latest Water Reuse Technologies Designed To Solve Global Water Scarcity Challenges. Water Online. https://www.wateron- line.com/doc/ge s-latest-water-reuse-technologies-designed-0001. October 2009.
77 Green to gold: how smart companies use environmental strategy to innovate, create value, and build competitive advantage. Daniel Esty and Andrew Winston. Hoboken, NJ: John Wiley & Sons. 2009.
78 Riding green wave, Philips says ' let there be LED'. Reuters. https://w ww.reuters.com/article/feature-philips-led/riding-gree n-wave-philips-say s-let-there-be-led-idUKLNE61801L20100209. February 2010.
79 Philips presents connected lighting for energy efficient and safer cities. Philips. https:// HYPERLINK http://www.philips.com/a-w/about/news/archive/ www.philips.com/a-w/about/news/archive/ standard/news/backgrounders/2014/2014 0331-Philips-presents-co nnected-lighting-fo r-energy-efficient-and-safer-cities.html. 2014.
80 Measuring Impact: How Business Accelerates the Sustainable Development Goals. UNDP and GRI. 2016.
81 Green to gold: how smart companies use environmental strategy to innovate, create value, and build competitive advan- tage. Daniel Esty and Andrew Winston. Hoboken, NJ: John Wiley & Sons. 2009.
82 Ibid.
83 Ibid.
84 Ibid.
85 How Smart Companies Use Environmental Strategy to Innovate, Create Value, and Build Competitive Advantage. Daniel C. Esty and Andrew S. Winston. New Haven: Yale University Press. 2006
86 Case Study: The Toyota Prius: Lessons in marketing eco-friendly products. Rudi Halbright and Max Dunn. http://www.maxdunn. com/stora ge/w w w.ma xdu n n.com/PM BA :%20Presid io%20 MBA%20Home/Prius Marketing Case Study.pdf. 2010.
87 Ibid.
88 How Smart Companies Use Environmental Strategy to Innovate, Create Value, and Build Competitive Advantage. Daniel C. Esty and Andrew S. Winston. New Haven: Yale University Press. 2006

89 Shared Value, Shared Responsibility: A Co-Creation Perspective on Sustainability. Sophie E. Andersen & Anne Ellerup Nielsen in Enterprising Initiatives in the Experience Economy: Transforming Social Worlds Edited by Britta Timm Knudsen, Dorthe Refslund Christensen, & Per Blenker
90 Green to gold: how smart companies use environmental strategy to innovate, create value, and build competitive advantage. Daniel Esty and Andrew Winston. Hoboken, NJ: John Wiley & Sons. 2009.
91 Nestle Invests $487 million in Sustainable Coffee Sourcing. Sustainable Brands. http://www.sustainablebrands.com/newsandviews/article s/nestle-invests-487-million-sustainable-coffee-sourcing. August 2010.
92 Nescafe Plan. Nescafe. https:// HYPERLINK http://www.nescafe.co.uk/nescafe-plan www.nescafe.co.uk/nescafe-plan. 2010.
93 The Walmart Sustainability Index FAQs. Walmart. HYPERLINK http://custom-/ http://custom- ers.icix.com/?wpfb dl=2 8.
94 The Business of Sustainability: McKinsey Global Survey Results. McKinsey & Company. 2012.
95 Sustainability's Next Frontier: Walking the Talk on the Sustainability Issues that Matter Most. MIT Sloan Management Review and The Boston Consulting Group. HYPERLINK http://sloanreview/ http://sloanreview.mit.edu/projects/sustainabilitys-next-frontier/. 2013
96 Ibid.
97 Ibid.
98 Triple Bottom Line as Sustainable Corporate Performance: A Proposition for the Future. Hasan Fauzi, Goran Svensson, and Azhar Abdul Rahman. Sustainability, 2(5), 1345-1360. 2010.
99 7 Companies Proving Triple Bottom Line Is Possible. Earth 911. https://earth911.com/business-policy/triple-bottom-line-7-companies/. August 2016.
100 Responsible Business Conduct: The OECD Guidelines for Multinational Enterprise. Business and Industry Advisory Committee to the OECD (BIAC). June 2015
101 Ibid.
102 Global Reporting Initiative. https://www.globalreporting.org/ Pages/default.aspx.
103 Sustainability Reporting Guidelines. Global Reporting Initiative. https://www.globalreporting.org/resourcelibrary/G3.1-Guidelines-Incl-Technical-Protocol.pdf. 2011.
104 Ibid.
105 GRI Sustainability Reporting: How valuable is the journey?. Global Reporting Initiative. https:// HYPERLINK http://www.globalreporting.org/resourceli- www.globalreporting.org/resourceli- brary/Starting-Points-2-G3.1.pdf. 2011.

106 How the G4 guidelines shape sustainability reporting. Chhavi Ghuliani, BSR. ht tps://w w w.greenbiz.com/ blog/2013/07/18/ g4-guidelines-futur e-sustainability-reporting. 2013
107 Highlights: GRI at 20. Global Reporting Initiative. https://HYPERLINK http://www.globalreporting.org/gri-2 www.globalreporting.org/gri-2 0/ Pages/Facts-and-figures.aspx. 2017.
108 The Integrated Reporting Movement: Meaning, Momentum, Motives, and Materiality. Robert G. Eccles, Michael P. Krzus, and Sydney Ribot. New Jersey: John Wiley & Sons Inc. 2015.
109 Achieving Sustainability Through Integrated Reporting. Robert G. Eccles & Daniela Saltzman. Stanford Social Innovation Review Summer 2011.
110 2016 One Report. Southwest Airlines. HYPERLINK http:// southwestonereport/ http://southwestonereport. com/2016/. 2016
111 CDL ups the game on integrated reporting in Singapore. Eco-Business. HYPERLINK http://www.eco-business.com/news/ cdl-ups-the-gam http://www.eco-business.com/news/cdl-ups-the-gam e-on-integrated-reporting-in-singapore/. May 2015
112 WBCSD website. HYPERLINK http://www.wbcsd.org/Overview/About-us http://www.wbcsd.org/Overview/About-us
113 Measuring Impact Framework Methodology. W B C S D & I F C . h t t p : / / d o c s . w b c s d . o r g / 2 017 / 01/ MeasuringImpactFrameworkMethodology. pdf. April 2008.
114 Ibid.
115 Ibid.
116 Measuring Impact: How Business Accelerates the Sustainable Development Goals. Business Call to Action (BCtA) and GRI. 2016.
117 The Business and Industr y's v ision and priorities for t he Sustainable Development Goals - Major Group Position Paper. United Nations. https:// sustainabledevelopment.un.org/content/ documents/3432SD2015%20 Position%20Paper Business%20&%20Industry.pdf. March 2014.
118 SDG Compass: The guide for business action on the SDGs. GRI, UN Global Compact & WBCSD. 2016.
119 Ibid.
120 Ibid.
121 What have the millennium development goals achieved? The Guardian. https://w w w.theguardian.com/global-development/ d at ablog /2015/ju l /0 6/what-m i l len n ium-de velopment-goal s-achieved-mdgs. 2015.
122 Embedding the Environment in Sustainable Development Goals. Post-2015 Discussion Paper 1. Version 1. https://sustain- abledevelopment.un.org/ content/documents/2037embedding-en- vironments-in-SDGs-v2.pdf. UNEP. July 2013.

123 Ibid.
124 Half of Weather Disasters Linked to Climate Change. National Geographic. HYPERLINK http://news.nationalgeographic.com/2015/11/15110 http://news.nationalgeographic.com/2015/11/15110 5-climate-weather-disasters-drought-storms/. 2015
125 Mainstreaming the 2030 Agenda for Sustainable Development: Interim Reference Guide to UN Country Teams. UN Development Group. ht t p://w w w.u ndp.org /c ontent/d a m /u ndp/ l ibr a r y/MDG/Post 2015-SDG/UNDP-SDG-U NDG-Reference-Guid e-UNCTs -2 015.pdf. 2015.
126 German Council for Sustainable Development. https://www.nachhaltigkeitsrat.de/en/the-council/fact-sheet/
127 Navigating the SDGs: a business guide to engaging with the UN Global Goals. PriceWaterhouse Coopers. 2016.
128 SDG Industry Matrix: Food, Beverage and Consumer Goods. February 2016
129 Navigating the SDGs: a business guide to engaging with the UN Global Goals. PriceWaterhouse Coopers. 2016.
130 Ibid.
131 Does corporate social responsibility affect the cost of capital? Sadok El Ghoul, Omrane Guedhami, Chuck C.Y. Kwok and Dev Mishra. Journal of Banking & Finance, 35(9). 2011.
132 Ibid.
133 Sustainability: CFOs are coming to the table. Deloitte. 2012.
134 BOP: a business strategy. Down to Earth. HYPERLINK http://downtoearth/ http://downtoearth. danone.com/2012/08/22/bop-a-business-strategy/. 2012
135 Net positive thinking in property. JLL. HYPERLINK http://w/ http://w w w.jll.co.uk /u nited-k ingdom/en-gb/news/3039/net-positive-t hink ing-in-property. April 2017.
136 Elephant Park. Lendlease. https:/ HYPERLINK http://www.lendlease.com/uk/projects/ /ww HYPERLINK http://www.lendlease.com/uk/projects/ w.lendlease.com/uk/projects/elephant-park/?id=3c8e138c-140a-4268-8cba-199afaec168d
137 Beyond carbon-neutral: What 'net positive' means for real estate. JLL. https://HYPERLINK http://www.jllrealviews.com/trends/beyond-carbon-neutra www.jllrealviews.com/trends/beyond-carbon-neutra l-what-net-positive-means-for-real-estate/. 2017
138 Going "net positive" is the next big thing on the sustainability agenda for real estate. Relx Group. https://sdgresources.relx.com/ articles/net-positive-thinking-property. 2017.
139 Ibid.
140 Towards Low GHG and Resilient Buildings. Global Alliance for Buildings and Construction. 2016.

141 Buildings and Climate Change Status, challenges, and opportu- nities. United Nations Environment Programme. 2007
142 Towards Low GHG and Resilient Buildings. Global Alliance for Buildings and Construction. 2016.
143 Environmental Sustainability Principles for the Real Estate Industry. World Economic Forum. January 2016.
144 Towards Low GHG and Resilient Buildings. Global Alliance for Buildings and Construction. 2016.
145 Environmental Sustainability Principles for the Real Estate Industry. World Economic Forum. January 2016.
146 Conserve as it constructs. Bloomberg. https://data.bloomber- glp.com/professional/sites/4/ESG CDL CASE BPS.pdf. 2016; Advancing Responsible Business Practices in Land, Construction and Real Estate Use and Investment. UN Global Compact. June 2015.
147 Environmental Sustainability Principles for the Real Estate Industry. World Economic Forum. January 2016.
148 W hat's in a Target? Investors Expect Signif ica nt Carbon Reductions from Real Estate Sector. GR ESB. ht tps://gresb. com/whats-target-investors-expec t-significant-carbon-reducti ons-real-estate-sector/. 2015

Chapter 3

Majid Al Futtaim: doing well by doing good

From 1995 in Deira, to MENA and beyond

Majid Al Futtaim is the leading shopping mall, communities, retail and leisure pioneer across the Middle East, Africa and Asia. In 2018, the revenue of the Company was US$ 9.5 billion a long way from 1995 when it all started with the establishment of the City Centre Deira and the adjoining Sofitel Hotel in Dubai (United Arab Emirates). Today, Majid Al Futtaim has a footprint in 15 countries.

The Company currently employs over 43,000 people and serves approximately 560 million visitors through its consumer offerings. It owns and operates 25 shopping malls, 13 hotels and four mixed-use communities, with further developments underway in the MENA region and beyond. In 2013, Majid Al Futtaim acquired full ownership of the Carrefour franchise in the region[149], and in 2017, the Company announced the acquisition of Retail Arabia, which entailed the rebranding of all Geant hypermarkets, supermarkets and convenience stores as Carrefour[150]. Majid Al Futtaim also operates 400 VOX Cinema screens and 36 Magic Planet family entertainment centers across the region, in addition to iconic leisure and entertainment facilities such as Ski Dubai and Ski Egypt, among others.

In fact, it is worth highlighting one of these key iconic developments, Ski Dubai, which demonstrates the uniqueness of the operations.

Located inside Mall of the Emirates in Dubai, Ski Dubai is the Middle East's first and the world's largest indoor ski resort (according to the Guinness Book of World Records) and indoor snow park. Ski Dubai spans over an area of 22,500 square meters with real snow, and offers snow-centered activities including skiing, snowboarding, tobogganing, meeting Gentoo and King penguins, or simply enjoying the sub-zero temperatures.[151] In 2017, Majid Al Futtaim opened a similar facility in Cairo, Egypt.[152]

In addition to being a pioneering player in developing world class communities and retail facilities, Majid Al Futtaim is the parent company to the consumer finance firm 'Najm', a fashion retail business representing international brands such as Abercrombie & Fitch, AllSaints, lululemon athletica, Crate & Barrel and Maison du Monde. In addition, Majid Al Futtaim operates Enova, a facility and energy management company, through a joint venture operation with Veolia, a global leader in optimized environment resource management. The Company also owns the rights to The LEGO Store and American Girl in the Middle East and operates in the food and beverage industry through a partnership with Gourmet Gulf. This is not an exhaustive list, but goes to show the diversity and depth of the business, and its geographical spread.

Majid Al Futtaim built strong corporate fundamentals over the years, reflected in its robust financial profile and steady growth. Between 2010 and 2015, revenues grew at a compounded annual growth rate of 10%, and asset holdings almost doubled in the same time period. The bulk of the revenue is generated through the UAE operations, followed by Saudi Arabia. The retail segment of the business is the main source of revenue (80%), followed by properties (13.2%) and ventures (6.8%). The Company is also the highest credit-rated privately owned corporate in the GCC region.

Currently, Majid Al Futtaim has several mall and hypermarket development projects in the pipeline in the UAE, Egypt, Oman, Saudi Arabia, Jordan, and Lebanon. Moving forward, it aims to protect its leadership position in its core countries and expand in adjacent geographical locations. Building a foundation position in African countries and expanding into diverse businesses are also strategic priorities for the Company in the medium to long term.

The first steps on the 1000-mile road to sustainability

Since inception, the Company's founder has been passionate about giving back to the community. This was, and still is, part of the Company's DNA. Over the years, passionate employees launched a number of community initiatives, and the Company provided all the support needed to introduce and run these initiatives.

While these were positive and welcome, it was clear to all that with the growth that is being delivered, and the impact on the societies it operates in, the Company needed to formalize its approach to being a responsible corporate citizen. As such, in 2010, corporate responsibility was prioritized and integrated in the Company's formal strategy.

With the launch of this strategy, the Company institutionalized and streamlined its CSR programme, and marked the ways in which the strategy would be embedded throughout the business divisions. Through stakeholder engagement and a detailed risk review, the strategy identified five areas of material impact:

(i) labor conditions and the supply chain
(ii) resource efficiency
(iii) employees
(iv) customers and tenants
(v) community and economic development

In each area, a set of targets were identified and performance was tracked against these targets over the years.

To ensure consistent and sustainable delivery, this was managed like any other strategic priority. A CSR governance structure was established and champions were identified and rewarded for their activities.

This was also supported by a wide-spread information campaign. In an effort to entrench CSR in the organizational culture and ensure that every employee understood the "what and why" of CSR at Majid Al Futtaim, a comprehensive plan of training and engagement for staff members was launched. This plan encompassed quarterly CSR breakfasts and a target to train hundreds of staff in corporate responsibility, green buildings and sustainability by the end of 2012.

This ambitious and transparent strategy was the start of a great journey as it built on the strength points in the business, and boldly addressed areas that required more focused attention. One of these areas was health and safety.

In implementing this strategy and its related metrics, the Company identified a number of challenges pertaining to health and safety. Local standards in the Company's countries of operations were well below global best practice - something that the teams started to tackle immediately, and with full management support. In 2011 – a year after the launch of this formal CSR strategy – Majid Al Futtaim achieved 78% of its CSR targets for the year. In 2012, this percentage rose to 84%[153]. These metrics were not only measured and monitored for the sake of internal management meetings, they were reported widely. This was a regional first in terms of transparency, openness, and commitment to improvement.

Having had some initial successes, and having identified the areas that needed improvement, Majid Al Futtaim took the focus on CSR to the next level. In 2013, the Company conducted an in-depth strategy and materiality review. This involved an analysis of its progress to date, consideration of individual country risks, and a review of what Majid Al Futtaim's peers were doing on CSR and sustainability. The review also included an examination of areas where opportunities exist to demonstrate leadership through innovation. This was the extent of the Company's focus - why be "good enough" when you can be a leader in the field!

The exercise was thorough, and engaged internal and external stakeholders to provide feedback on the sustainability impacts the stakeholders considered to be most important for the business. As a result of this review, a range of issues were refined and a new five-year sustainability strategy was formulated.

This new approach aimed to establish pioneering standards across Majid Al Futtaim, and to develop and manage high performance assets that support prosperous communities. The Company moved from CSR as a focus, to sustainability as a strategic priority. Those first steps in 2010 became a way of life today.

In fact, the Majid Al Futtaim Chief Executive Officer Alain Bejjani continually refers to sustainability as a necessity. "It is undeniable that the world today is faced with environmental challenges more than ever before. With natural resources depleting at an alarming pace, sustainability is no longer just an aspiration; it is a necessity".

The strategy was designed to be supported by strong foundations for embedding sustainability policies. These included the latest thinking and practice in the domain covering:

- green building policy
- energy management policy
- health and safety standards
- labor conditions standards
- pre-acquisition checklists

Long term goals, which were supported by annual targets, and "big ideas" that were to be set and driven through employee engagement were also embedded into this sustainability strategy.

Once the strategy was set, and the ambition confirmed, the hard work began. There were lots of challenges when it came to implementation.

The most prominent of which was the talent and skills needed for such a forward-looking sustainability agenda. The specialized human resources that could design specific policies (e.g. health and safety policy) were a critical gap, leading to slow progress in some areas. This was not a unique situation with the Company itself, but indeed a reflection of the skills and practices in the markets it operated in. These skills were underdeveloped, in general, and not much in demand. Needless to say, this triggered major investments in the Company's human capital.

Reducing energy consumption and waste generation in the Company's malls was also an area that required more focused attention - something that all companies working in the real estate sector in the Middle East faced. This was a novel concept in the region, in many ways ahead of local and regional public regulations, and building on an old legacy system that did not prioritize these matters. Making the existing built environment eco-friendlier, and moving from incremental to substantial environmental improvements was, and still remains, a sector-wide challenge[154].

Moreover, and possibly more challenging than making the Company's own infrastructure more sustainable, was influencing tenant behavior and convincing them to move towards more sustainable consumption. Majid Al Futtaim's tenants account for more than half the company's operational environmental impact and getting them on board was key.

To ensure that they were aligned with the Company's vision for sustainability, Majid Al Futtaim introduced a pioneering initiative called the Green Star Rating programme in 2012. This was intended to be a compelling tool to drive greener retail operations that assessed the sustainability credentials of store fit-outs at Majid Al Futtaim-owned shopping malls. However, an evaluation of the programme in the City Centre Beirut mall in 2013 showed that among the 170 tenants audited, only three achieved a Green Star Rating. Further analysis revealed that the low level of Green Star Ratings was owing to a complex submission process and lack of engagement with tenants prior to fit-out. Many lessons were learnt. These feedback loops have been crucial in the sustainability journey, and have led to critical, and incremental improvements that helped the Company reach the stage it is at today. The rating system has been widely adopted across the Company's malls, and currently 638 stores belonging to 254 parent companies are rated 3 stars or above.

Another challenge that the Company was faced with was data. Evaluating environmental impact across the whole value chain was a tall task. Environmental data management systems were in a nascent phase and needed to be strengthened to better measure and monitor the gains made in energy and water usage and waste. A methodology needed to be put into place to assess the socio-economic impacts of Majid Al Futtaim's portfolio. Internal processes had to be developed and refined to ensure the continued embedding of sustainability across the Company and within the day-to-day working of its staff[155].

Sustainability as an organizational system

Despite some initial operational and cultural challenges, Majid Al Futtaim made progress towards the three-year goals that were set at the onset of its CSR efforts. Between 2010 and 2013, the Company granted more than US$ 8 million in cash or in-kind support to local community initiatives and made significant improvements to the living conditions of contractor workers across its supply chain. It also performed 96 labor accommodation audits, and provided sustainability training to hundreds of employees over this time period. In 2013, Majid Al Futtaim achieved 91% of its targets (66% were fully achieved and 25% partially achieved).

In terms of community and economic development, in 2013 alone, the Company undertook community investment worth more than US$ 3 million. An employee volunteering programme was also launched in the same year, and the internship programme was expanded to include job shadowing placements for local young people in UAE, Bahrain, Egypt, Oman and Lebanon. On the operational consumption level, energy and water consumption in like-for-like portfolio was reduced by 3% and 4%, respectively.

To further build its own knowledge base, networks, and transfer of know-how, a sustainability summit was held to gather global experts to discuss important sustainability issues affecting the Middle East region, and to build relationships between all those involved in delivering sustainability at Majid Al Futtaim.

In that three-year period (2010-2013), Majid Al Futtaim achieved two thirds of its resource efficiency targets including a 19.9% reduction in hotel energy consumption on a 2009 baseline. This was over and above the set target of 15%. More importantly, 'Green' clauses were added in all new tenancy agreements since 2011 and by the end of 2013, 100% of leases had such clauses. These clauses committed Majid Al Futtaim and its tenants to work together to reduce adverse environmental impacts.

The continuous improvement of labor conditions within Majid Al Futtaim and across the value chain was also prioritized. The aim was to continually improve the lives of laborers and migrant workers and enhance the quality of service that Majid Al Futtaim's contractors delivered.

Starting with the basics of health and safety, Majid Al Futtaim recorded zero fatalities in 2013, with more than 11 million hours worked on construction sites. That was the goal, and always remains the key target. In the same period, overall accident frequency rate among direct employees and contractors dropped by a third. For example, the accident frequency rate for Oman and UAE fell to 1.69 accidents per 100,000 employee hours worked - down from 2.61 in 2012. This was all possible with a structured system, and management commitment; 61 health and safety audits were conducted in 2013.

Some further gains were made to improve living conditions for contractor employees who live in staff accommodation working on Majid Al Futtaim's assets and developments. Between 2010 and 2013, Majid Al Futtaim conducted 96 staff accommodation audits in a bid to drive improvements across the Company's supplier base and ensure they remain in line with international best practice. In 2014, a new labour conditions policy was launched, which set out commitments to safeguard worker rights across all developments, including timely remuneration, annual leave and accommodation standards.

In that year (2014), Majid Al Futtaim achieved the highest 'Green Star' status with the Global Real Estate Sustainability Benchmark (GRESB), which compares 637 real estate companies globally on a range of measures from energy reduction performance to the quality of their sustainability policies.

However, there were some areas where Majid Al Futtaim was not able to meet its sustainability targets. Between 2010 and 2013, the number of spot checks at assets led by senior officials lagged behind the committed target. The aim of these director-led spot checks was to raise awareness of conditions across the business, and emphasize the importance of audits to contractors. In 2015, Majid Al Futtaim conducted a gap analysis of the health and safety measures taken across the business. This analysis revealed that while some business units were making significant strides towards alignment with OHSAS 18001 best practice standards on health and safety management, other parts were not as advanced. To address this, the Company appointed a health and safety manager to oversee the construction side of the business, a step towards defining clear ownership of health and safety issues for the first time. In 2018, Majid Al Futtaim implemented its Health and Safety Policy.

Majid Al Futtaim also struggled in the areas of reducing energy and water consumption and attaining recycling targets, especially in its operational malls. These challenges produced useful lessons, and all of them were tackled in future years. It is key to note however, that they are a constant reminder of the bumpy road to achieving such ambitious targets.

By the year 2015, a lot of the sustainability practices and culture have become institutionalized. When Majid Al Futtaim inaugurated the City Centre Me'aisem mall in Dubai in September 2015, the mall became the first development in the Middle East to achieve LEED Platinum status for green buildings (within two months of opening). The LEED (Leadership in Energy and Environmental Design) accreditation system, which is the most widely used third-party verification for green buildings around the world, ranks developments across various sustainability criteria, including water use and energy efficiency. Platinum certification at City Centre Me'aisem, which hosts 54 shops across 31,200 square meters, came about because the development secured 80 points out of a possible 110 available across all criteria.

Among the innovative measures that helped to achieve platinum status was the use of materials that reflect heat away from the mall and reduce the heat island effect, where the mall can become significantly warmer than the surrounding area because of solar gain. This material was used on more than 75% of the roof area. Points were also scored for the widespread use of materials – such as paints, coatings, adhesives and sealants – that contained a low volume of Volatile Organic Compounds (VOCs) content, providing a healthier interior environment. Furthermore, an indoor air quality management plan was implemented on the construction site to protect workers. There was also a waste management plan that helped to divert waste away from landfill during construction, and an environmental management plan that ensured more general protection of the environment. Car park shading structures at the mall have integrated solar panels that generate 12% of the annual energy consumption of the entire building, which also uses low energy LED lighting throughout. All of the water needed for irrigation is provided by an onsite treatment plant that recycles grey water from the mall's washrooms.

Sustainability has become a natural way of doing business in Majid Al Futtaim.

Raising the bar: introducing Net Positive

In 2014, an organization-wide sustainability review was conducted. While the developments thus far had been significant and exciting, there was scope for the Company to innovate and do more in the sustainability realm. With the aim of integrating sustainability as a critical element of the Company's future, the Net Positive ambition was launched. Carbon and Water were identified as the most crucial sustainability material issues and impact areas, therefore becoming the focus of the Company's Net Positive ambition.

This was the start of an exciting and a very technically challenging journey.

The organization-wide sustainability review prioritized a total of 26 material sustainability issues from a universe of 49 wider material sustainability issues. This prioritization was done in a very systemic manner and was based on:

- peer review
- baseline data assessment
- debt market expectations
- UNGC commitments
- internal risk registers, and
- sustainability market risk review.

To identify the issues for Net Positive impact from amongst these sustainability issues, Majid Al Futtaim applied two criteria. Firstly, it must be feasible to measure and quantify the impacts of the issue. In order for a material sustainability issue to be included as part of the Net Positive approach, Majid Al Futtaim must be able to measure and quantify the performance of the constituent material issues. This needed to be a data-driven policy.

Secondly, it must be possible to have a positive impact that goes beyond being 'neutral or 'zero', i.e. the sum of the positive impacts of an issue must be able to outweigh the sum of the negative impacts.

Having applied these criteria to the full list of material issues, it was determined that there are four potential impact areas in which Majid Al Futtaim could seek to achieve Net Positive:

1. Water
2. Carbon
3. Material Use
4. Social

These four areas were further assessed from the perspective of peer adoption, measurability of impact, and significance of impact in the region and globally. In this assessment, Carbon and Water emerged as the two impact areas that Majid Al Futtaim should focus on in its Net Positive approach.

In order to understand the feasibility and establish the scope of its Net Positive objectives, it was imperative for the Company to analyze its value chain and understand where impacts arise. Therefore, extensive research on carbon emissions and water consumption was conducted to assess the impact of the Company's managed and corporate assets. This had to be done in a structured way and assets were categorized according to business units, namely:

- Majid Al Futtaim - Retail
- Majid Al Futtaim - Properties
- Majid Al Futtaim - Ventures
    1. Fashion
    2. Leisure & Entertainment
    3. Finance
    4. Enova

With regard to both carbon and water, the research evaluated carbon emissions and water consumption in three separate impact areas (upstream, downstream, and operational impacts) within the value chain. The research also explored trade-offs between cost, difficulty of implementation, and Majid Al Futtaim's sphere of influence in each impact area at every stage of the value chain.

Carbon

In the carbon arena, Majid Al Futtaim's environmental data calculations showed that the Company's total carbon footprint amounted to 1,166,177 tonnes of CO_2 in 2015. Based on these calculations, Majid Al Futtaim set a target of reducing operational emissions from sources owned or controlled by Majid Al Futtaim (representing 61.2% of the Company's total carbon footprint) and target these emissions in the Net Positive strategy from 2017 onwards, while downstream emissions should be a secondary priority and should be targeted in the Net Positive strategy from 2020 onwards.[156]

Upstream emissions were to be excluded from Net Positive targets, as an upstream Net Positive carbon strategy would be complicated and expensive to implement, and only accounted for 25.1% of Majid Al Futtaim's total value chain emissions during 2015. Within operational emissions, the study recommended that the Company should primarily focus on carbon reductions and energy improvements within the Retail and Properties businesses as they represent 86% of Majid Al Futtaim's total operational emissions, while the Leisure & Entertainment businesses should be secondary concerns. Moreover, with regard to energy efficiency, the report proposed that Majid Al Futtaim should identify 'easy wins' within its operations (for example switching to low energy lighting or turning non-essential electrical system off standby).

Water

Majid Al Futtaim's portfolio had an estimated water footprint of 45,060,041 m 3 in 2015 from water consumed over its entire value chain. The research revealed the greatest source of water consumption arose from the upstream impact area, which represented 86.2% of the value chain. However, due to Majid Al Futtaim's limited influence over upstream consumption, the sustainability review recommended that this area should be excluded from the Net Positive targets. Operational consumption, which represented 12.4% of total water footprint, should remain the focus of attention in Majid Al Futtaim's Net Positive strategy from 2017 onwards, as the Company's high level of influence over operations could ensure that sustainable change was achievable, verifiable and cost-effective. Within operational consumption, the study recommended that the Net Positive strategy should emphasize water reductions within the Retail and Properties businesses (which constitute 84% of total water consumption), with secondary focus on water reductions within the Leisure & Entertainment businesses. Water reductions at Enova, Finance and Fashion businesses should not be included in the Net Positive targets.

Downstream water impacts (constituting 1.4% of water footprint) were to be a secondary priority, and reducing water consumption in this area would be challenging as it is the responsibility of tenants which Majid Al Futtaim has a limited influence over. Thus, downstream impacts were to be included in the Net Positive strategy from 2020 onwards.

Once launched, the strategy was well-received by the Company's stakeholders. Not only was this the first of its kind in the region, it was also fully aligned with national commitments that the United Arab Emirates (where Majid Al Futtaim is headquartered) has made, both locally and internationally. The UAE Minister of Climate Change and Environment, Dr. Thani Al Zeyoudi, noted that "Majid Al Futtaim's Net Positive commitment is a landmark step in helping to create a more sustainable future for our region. The strategy is in line with the UAE Green Agenda and the UAE National Climate Change Plan to address solutions to pressing current and future environmental challenges. Collaboration with the private sector is key to realizing our sustainability goals and promoting a shared responsibility for our environment".

In data we trust: establishing a baseline for Net Positive

In order to define the scope of Net Positive for Majid Al Futtaim, establishing the level of control over various aspects of carbon and water footprints as well as the quality and availability of data was a vital task. The Company used a systematic approach (illustrated below) to determine material issues and component parts, and finalize which issues were to be included within the scope of Net Positive commitments and targets.

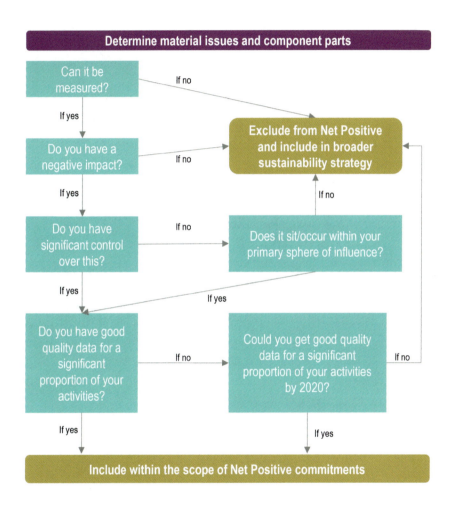

With regard to operational carbon emissions, Majid Al Futtaim broke down operational carbon footprint by country. This revealed that UAE operations accounted for 55.5% of the carbon footprint. An advantage in this context was that UAE is both the area where Majid Al Futtaim has most influence in, and the Company has the best availability of energy data in the region, particularly in relation to forecasting towards 2030.

The next step was to conduct a scenario analysis. This was done based on two energy production and grid decarbonization policies/targets in the UAE[1], which were estimated to reduce emissions by 15% by 2030. The UAE scenarios were applied to emissions from all countries where Majid Al Futtaim operates, with the assumption that grid decarbonization would be similar throughout the whole MENA region. The scale of the challenge for Majid Al Futtaim was depicted through these scenario analyses, and an estimate of carbon reductions between 2015 and 2030 was calculated. This estimate allowed the Company to identify its Net Positive targets, i.e. the emissions remaining after the 15% reduction was achieved through decarbonization in both scenarios.

In order to illustrate the financial implications of this scale of Net Positive projects, costs of two different routes (namely, renewables and offsetting) were assessed. These estimates and cost analyses enabled the definition of the direction of carbon Net Positive efforts, which were to focus on operational emissions as well as the sub-metered tenant consumption as these are the areas within the primary sphere of influence.

A similar approach was adopted to identify the direction of the Company in identifying water Net Positive commitments. A country breakdown revealed that UAE operations accounted for 55.2% of the water usage, which was comparable to the distribution of carbon emissions. The issues of water desalination and carbon intensity were

---

[1] Two scenarios were used for this analysis. The 2030 Reference Case (the most pessimistic scenario), which is based on existing and proposed energy developments, and REmap 2030, (the most optimistic case), which is based on IRENA's (International Renewable Energy Agency) realistic potential calculations for countries to scale up renewables.

also taken into consideration. A thorough cost analysis pointed towards focusing Net Positive efforts on the operational water footprint as well as the sub-metered tenant consumption, as these are the areas within the primary sphere of influence. Furthermore, it showed that while water desalination is a key Net Positive project for water, it has an associated carbon footprint that should be considered when measuring the carbon footprint going forward.

Next, the Company identified the impact areas for inclusion in the Net Positive efforts within the broader focus areas, i.e. Carbon and Water. To determine the impact areas for inclusion in the scope of Majid Al Futtaim's carbon Net Positive strategy, different carbon emissions' sources were ranked according to the Greenhouse Gas Protocol reporting principles. This exercise allowed the Company to further visualize the scale of the challenge and to exclude various items based on relevance, completeness, consistency, transparency and accuracy. To carry out impact area analysis, Majid Al Futtaim's carbon footprint was split into Majid Al Futtaim Properties and other business units. A ranking of various carbon emissions sources based on the Greenhouse Gas Protocol reporting principles for Majid Al Futtaim Properties was produced. This ranking allowed earmarking high priority and implementable areas.

This exercise enabled Majid Al Futtaim to understand what operational data is relatively easy to collect with good coverage and accuracy. Building emission data is readily available and can be collected using existing approaches. Downstream building emissions are also readily available with good coverage from tenant sub-meters, whereas tenant meters may require some tenant engagement. The biggest challenge was obtaining good quality upstream emissions data and it was found that the majority of it would have to be estimated. A similar evaluation was conducted for all other parts of the business that typically posed a higher initial challenge as less data has been collected at the time (especially for upstream emissions) and some of the values used were based on available benchmarks.

To ensure continuity and consistent methodology, the same approach was used for identifying impact areas for water, and the GHG Reporting Principles were leveraged to highlight priority areas. In addition, the ISO 14046:2014 standard principles were also used to establish a robust water footprint for Majid Al Futtaim. Similar to carbon data, downstream developments, refurbishments and fit-outs data is more difficult to obtain, particularly for the supply chain. As a result of data availability and level of control Majid Al Futtaim has, the Company decided on including operational building use, operational developments and downstream sub-metered water data into the scope of Net Positive.

For Majid Al Futtaim's other business units, the upstream data had to predominantly be estimated based on spend figures, which did not provide an accurate representation of the true values. Downstream data was easier to obtain, however required some degree of tenant engagement.

After this baseline analysis, the Company decided to include the full operational carbon and water footprints and downstream sub-metered tenant carbon and water footprints as well as the footprints arising from any Net Positive projects into the scope of Majid Al Futtaim's Net Positive strategy.

What can be measured, can be managed: measuring Net Positive

As a first step in its Net Positive journey, Majid Al Futtaim planned to define and measure its water and carbon impacts, and in that context, some principles were set out for measuring Net Positive. These principles have been devised by the Forum of the Future and are as follows:

1. Transparency: Majid Al Futtaim will publish its Net Positive methodology, detailing specifically the scope of its Net Positive approach.

2. Consistency: Majid Al Futtaim will capture all data with regards to its impact areas, both positive and negative impacts.

3. Completeness: Majid Al Futtaim will report the level of detail to which data is recorded and where data has been estimated. It will also report on what data it intends to record and what data it deems as immaterial.

4. Different Types of Impact will be kept separate: Majid Al Futtaim will develop separate Net Positive balances for both Water and Carbon impacts, so that positive impacts in one area are not traded off against negative impacts in another area.

5. Existing methods will be used where possible: Majid Al Futtaim will, as far as possible, use existing methodologies and protocols for calculating its total impacts.

6. Sharing data is vital: Majid Al Futtaim will regularly disclose the lessons it has learnt from Net Positive projects and reduction initiatives.

With these principles firmly in place, the Company needed to set out a clear methodology for measuring Net Positive commitments in each impact area. For each impact area, this methodology was employed:

- Defined Net Positive
- Identified which metrics will need to be used in the calculation of the impact; and
- Identified how to measure total impacts

This methodology is outlined in this section along the two distinct impact areas: carbon and water.

A) Carbon

The Forum for the Future provided a clear definition of being Net Positive in carbon: *"Being Net Positive in carbon means removing or avoiding the generation of more carbon than you create in your operations and/or across your value chain."*

For Majid Al Futtaim, being Net Positive implies that it must measure impacts, reduce impacts, and create positive impacts. To measure impact, Majid Al Futtaim plans to calculate a total carbon footprint using well established protocols and guidelines. Next, the Company will undertake reasonable steps to reduce its carbon emissions within its scope of activity. Finally, creating positive impact will entail delivering projects which will avoid emissions in areas outside of scope of activity. Thus, Majid Al Futtaim will define Net Positive Carbon as a state when emissions avoided by external projects outweigh the emissions that are generated as a result of Majid Al Futtaim's activities.

As for calculating the carbon impact, that would require Majid Al Futtaim to collect a variety of energy data points from both renewable and non-renewable sources. Majid Al Futtaim already measured a significant number of 'impact elements' using a number of metrics that are defined in the reporting guidelines set out by the Global Reporting Initiative (GRI) and the European Public Real Estate Association (EPRA).

However, the Company needed to begin measuring its energy consumption from both renewable and non-renewable sources. From this data, Majid Al Futtaim would be able to calculate the emissions using different methodologies for each metric.

B) Water

According to the Forum for the Future, being Net Positive in water means *"...helping to create more accessible water and better-quality water than you consume across your operations or your value chain."*

For Majid Al Futtaim to be seen as Net Positive in water, the Company needs to measure impacts by calculating its total water footprint, take steps to reduce the water footprint, and undertake projects that create more accessible water or better-quality water to the regions from where it has been extracted, or similarly water scarce regions. Thus, being Net Positive in water will imply that the water replenished / improved by external projects is more than the water consumed from main supplies.

Similar to carbon, a range of water metrics was available to be used to report in line with EPRA and GRI. In order to calculate each of the recommended water impact metrics, a number of methodologies were applied. These methodologies varied from metric to metric, and were tailored according to the impact metric under consideration. For example, while both measure impact on water metrics, the methodology that measures the amount of water recycled cannot be the same as the methodology measuring water which has been made accessible by a project.

Once it has identified specific metrics and methodologies to measure impact, Majid Al Futtaim will work on developing and delivering specific Net Positive projects which have measurable positive impacts. Ultimately, these positive impacts will outweigh any negative impacts from the business and therefore deliver a Net Positive benefit.

It is recognized that certain projects may be delivered that will have a positive impact but that cannot be measured and therefore will not contribute to individual Net Positive impact areas. Majid Al Futtaim is not doing all this as a number crunching exercise. It is part of how the Company views its impact on any region it operates in. Hussain Saqer, the General Manager of Sustainability in Majid Al Futtaim - Retail captured this spirit when he noted *"I hope our customers feel proud of our efforts to ensure a sustainable future which goes beyond the walls of our retail stores. We want to be a part of the communities in which we operate so our Net Positive commitment is a commitment to their future as much as it is to ours."*

From measuring to managing: organizational and operational change

Over the course of a Net Positive 'journey' ahead, it is anticipated that organizational and structural changes will occur within Majid Al Futtaim, like any other dynamic and growing firm. These may include situations involving the acquisition of subsidiary businesses and mergers with other businesses, and many other forms of organizational change. In order to ensure that these changes do not affect the Net Positive commitments, Majid Al Futtaim has put in place a number of processes and governance mechanisms to manage such occurrences. We call this managing forward.

This is a robust system, that is based on structured scenario planning for eventualities such as the sale/acquisition/development/demolition of assets, corporate office growth, and diversification of products and locations. Processes have been developed to ensure that each event is properly dealt with in terms of the Company's overall Net Positive approach.

Achieving Net Positive commitments by 2040 entails a dedicated and organized effort to design and implement relevant projects. To this end, a detailed implementation plan was put in place by Majid Al Futtaim to ensure that Net Positive is managed just like any other business imperative with the same rigor, focus, and resources.

In this broader implementation plan, the specific action plans for carbon and water have been divided into three sections based on the three-pronged approach to achieve Net Positive:

1. Measure impacts: Continually calculating the total water and carbon footprints of assets

2. Reduce negative impacts: projects to reduce carbon emissions and water consumption at assets
3. Create positive impacts: projects external to Majid Al Futtaim operations which will avoid emissions and create more accessible water or better quality water to the regions from where it has been extracted

This is all phase 1 of the Net Positive journey, wherein the Company's Net Positive approach was finalized and launched. With regard to the framework, the targets for each business were getting implemented and progress was reviewed against these targets annually. Moreover, initial communications were produced and Majid Al Futtaim plans to publish the results against announced targets annually. Staff training and capacity building activities were also being rolled out in this phase. Major efforts were also undertaken to shape the narrative. Majid Al Futtaim's sustainability team believe that to make Net Positive successful, it is important that the organization at large speaks one language and that the sustainability journey is translated into a simple story.

In the future, the Company will roll out phases 2 and 3. Progress will continue to be reviewed and human capital development will be ongoing. To ensure that its initiatives and efforts are relevant and effectively address pressing issues in sustainability, the Company will continuously review (and revise, where necessary) its strategy to ensure that it achieves its Net Positive targets by 2040.

Creating a Net Positive Impact will require significant input, co-operation and understanding from the whole company in each phase of the process. In the coming years, Majid Al Futtaim aims to reduce its operational impacts not just in carbon emissions and water consumption, but also in terms of wider impacts within the communities in which the Company operates. For this to be implemented efficiently, dedicated efforts are required in three key areas namely governance, data management and risk management.

In terms of governance, and in order to manage its Net Positive commitment, Majid Al Futtaim established governance structures that enable organization-wide change to come about. This included the creation of a Net Positive steering group that draws representation from all subsidiaries, and from executive leadership to help guide the implementation of initiatives. This group reports to the Majid Al Futtaim Board, where Net Positive is a regular agenda item. Moreover, the following resourcing mechanisms is leveraged to catalyze Net Positive strategy and initiatives, and monitor their progress:

1. <u>Board level sponsors</u> – across each subsidiary, a board level sponsor was identified. These sponsors maintain a deep level of understanding of the Net Positive aims and progress on action.

2. <u>Net Positive manager</u> – a full-time resource who sits within Majid Al Futtaim to support the business units and to oversee and manage all Net Positive programmes and action plans across all business units.

3. <u>Net Positive champions</u> – across each business, Majid Al Futtaim identified Net Positive champions who act as on-the-ground representatives to engage with colleagues and stakeholders on all matters relating to Majid Al Futtaim's Net Positive ambitions. These champions are assigned key targets, which are incorporated into their formal job descriptions (and/or annual Net Positive KPIs included as part of their annual performance review) so there is a sense of priority and value to their work on Net Positive.

On the data management front, the work ahead is much more critical, and much harder. The timely collection of accurate data is a critical success factor for the Net Positive journey. The information collected has to be managed and stored in an organized and retrievable manner. Data management systems will need to be strengthened significantly to manage the achievement of Net Positive commitments. Majid Al Futtaim is investing in the development of data management infrastructure as well as the professional development of staff that is involved in collecting and using the data to further the Net Positive agenda. Individuals with data collection responsibility have been identified in order to ensure that the data collected is accurate and complete. To ensure that information improves strategic decision-making, the Company is working to design a robust data management system, which will enable the development of efficient workflow management processes, safely store and manage large amounts of data over time. Moreover, it will also allow property and business managers to track projects and initiatives that will support the implementation of Majid Al Futtaim's Net Positive programme.

Lastly, the journey needs a robust risk management approach. The Company is working to identify risks emerging from all segments of stakeholders – customers, tenants, community, and staff. The main risks or challenges that Majid Al Futtaim expects to be faced with are the capacity of its staff to conceive Net Positive programmes and initiatives, measure impact, and implement these projects. In order to mitigate these risks from day 1, the Company started to undertake extensive training and professional development on an organization- wide basis. Training programmes aim to educate and familiarize team members with the principles of Net Positive and Majid Al Futtaim's focus areas and aims in each impact area. The conceptualization of projects will need to take a two-pronged approach – bottom-up combined with top-down. To ensure that projects are relevant and effectively rolled out, staff engagement and input will be a key contributing factor.

Given that the renewable energy landscape is still nascent in the MENA region, access to sources or suppliers of renewable energy can be a potential challenge for Majid Al Futtaim. In order to be Net Positive, the Company will need to engage with utility providers to invest in renewable energy. The decline in oil prices, and the MENA governments' push towards renewable energy are likely to further the Company's agenda in this respect as an increasing number of utility providers are looking to invest in renewable energy sources in the MENA region today compared to earlier years.

All these risks notwithstanding, the Net Positive strategy has been approved, delivered, and now gone into implementation. The journey to Net Positive has started, the leadership is behind it, the mindset has changed, and Majid Al Futtaim is setting an example in the region. This lighthouse strategy will have much wider benefits to the whole region, beyond the abstract numbers in the Company, which are going to be impressive in their own right. For Majid Al Futtaim, there is no looking back, and the future is Net Positive.

(Endnotes)

149 Majid Al Futtaim acquires full ownership of Carrefour franchise in the region. Gulf News. May 11, 2013. HYPERLINK http://gulfnews.com/ http://gulfnews.com/ business/sectors/investment/majid-al-futtaim-acquires-ful l-ow nership-of-carrefour-franchise-in-the-region-1.1187332

150 Majid Al Futtaim buys Geant franchise owner in region. GulfNews. June 29, 2017. HYPERLINK http://gulfnews.com/business/sectors/retail/majid-a http://gulfnews.com/business/sectors/retail/majid-a l-futtaim-buys-geant-franchise-owner-in-region-1.2050679

151 Ski Dubai. Majid Al Futtaim. http://www.majidal-futtaim.com/our-businesses/leisure-entertainment/unique-leisure-destinations/ski-dubai

152 Snow time like the present: Cairo gets its own indoor ski park. Arab News. HYPERLINK http://w/ http://w ww.arabnews.com/node/1063976/corporate-news. March 6th, 2017.

153 Majid Al Futtaim Corporate Social Responsibility Report 2011

154 Cha l lenges for Susta inabi lit y Innovat ions in Rea l Estate a nd Construction Industr y. Ju ho-Kusti Kaja nderl, Mat ti Siv unen, Ju k ka Heinonen, and Seppo Junnila. Paper pre- sented at LCM 2011. HYPERLINK http://www.lcm2011.org/papers.html?- http://w w w.lcm2011.org/papers.html?- file=tl files/pdf/paper/3 Session LCM Tools%20for Green a n d Su s t a i n ab le B u i l d i n gs/ 1 K aj a n d e r- Challenges for Sustainability Innovations-728 b.pdf

155 Majid Al Futtaim Sustainability Report 2013 – Transforming Tomorrow

156 Our Net Positive Commitment White Paper. Majid Al Futtaim. 2017.

Chapter 4

A blueprint for Net Positive: helping businesses give more than they take

Beyond the environmental standards and toward a shared environment

Increasing demand for food, water, energy and minerals is putting greater pressure on the planet. Over the next decade, trillions of dollars will be invested in mining and energy development, much of it in undeveloped natural areas. The future sustainability of these places depends on making better decisions now about how we protect, manage, and develop our lands and waters.

Conserving global biodiversity without compromising economic development is a defining challenge of the 21st century. Today, and in light of the unprecedented global decline in biological diversity, the world is waking up to the fact that attainment of sustainable development goals is inextricably linked to more effective and responsible management of biodiversity. Businesses, which rely on everything from fresh water to protection from natural disasters, are recognizing that they need to look at the big picture – how their activities are linked to biodiversity and ecosystem services – in order to thrive, and the number of businesses that are setting more targeted and measurable environmental goals, and making commitments to achieving a net positive impact on biodiversity, is increasing.

Indeed, around the globe, net positive is becoming the new target for many companies. Not simply a corporate social responsibility exercise, but the way they would like to do business. As the effects of climate change become more visible in our everyday lives, businesses realize that this is not a matter that should be left for the government to handle alone. This is a whole-of-society matter, and one that we should all work together to solve, as entities and individuals. Businesses are also realizing that not addressing environmental sustainability can result in resource constraints, supply chain risks, branding mishaps, and alienation of customers. So, the issue of a triple bottom line is now becoming a core element of business strategy. Many are now emphasizing sustainability in a way that extends beyond reducing the negative impact, and aiming at the creation of positive social value as a priority, over and above the simple adherence to minimum environmental standards and policies. Indeed, it is very encouraging to see more and more companies aiming to have a net positive environmental footprint while also generating a positive impact on their bottom line. This is the start of new era in how we do business, perceive the business role in society, and how we manage our environment.

However, in order to become net positive, businesses have to address a number of philosophical and practical concerns. Some of these concerns relate to the Company's contextual definition of net positive and the impacts that should be taken into consideration. Once this is defined clearly, companies have to decide how the impacts should be measured, compared and communicated.

They do this with a clear focus on the big picture of a sustainable healthy planet, and with an eye on business benefits. Indeed, it has been demonstrated that businesses who take a proactive approach to managing their environmental impact and demonstrate to stakeholders that they can deliver on sustainability targets are likely to have several competitive advantages, including:

- Access to land and resources – a reputation for strong environmental management increases the likelihood of a business being granted access to land by governments, and of attracting partners, employees and customers.

- Access to finance – given tightening standards of financial institutions, a company that has a commitment to, and delivers on net positive will be more likely to gain access to finance from entities like the International Finance Corporation (IFC), the Equator Banks and other similar financial institutions.
- License to operate – strong environmental practices can boost a business's reputation with regulators, local communities and civil society, and can improve relationships with stakeholders who are affected by a company's impact on ecosystem services.
- Operational cost effectiveness – by integrating ecosystem services into business, companies can avoid compliance costs, fines and legal fees and minimize costs for resources such as freshwater.
- Operational stability – by reducing potentially negative impacts on those ecosystem services upon which a company's operations depend, the medium and long-term sustainability of those operations is ensured.

Given that each company's vision, offerings and processes are different, there is no one-size-fits-all approach to becoming Net Positive. Nevertheless, the motivation to achieve net positive outcomes is consistent, and all businesses aiming to become net positive must integrate a set of net positive principles to design a robust approach to achieve their vision.

The aim of this section of the book is to offer a practical blueprint to help companies start their net positive journey.

Net Positive Principles

While the net positive movement is building momentum, it remains an emerging concept. There is a lot of experimentation going on, and no one "wrote the guidebook" yet. In this context, it is important to start with the basics. For those companies who want to embark on a net positive journey, it is critical to accept, at the outset, that this is a marathon, not a sprint. More importantly, it is a marathon along new routes that are still emerging.

Having said that, the destination for all these new routes is the same: to become thriving organizations that deliver benefits that extend far beyond traditional organizational boundaries.

Having accepted that, it is also important to accept that this will require risk taking, and a lot of innovation. Becoming net positive requires organizations to be ambitious and plan for long-term success. They have to go beyond risk avoidance and incremental improvements and start to innovate.

While there are no specific guidelines for the next steps, there is a general set of principles that can guide this journey. The following is a description of the core ones.

		Net Positive Principles
1.	Material Impact	The organization has a clear objective to have a positive impact in its key material areas.
2.	Evidence	The positive impact of a business's Net Positive efforts should be clearly demonstrable, even if it cannot be measured accurately.
3.	Best Practice	While the aim to be Net Positive in its key material areas is essential, the organization should also demonstrate best practice in corporate responsibility and sustainability across its economic, social and environmental impact areas. Moreover, these best practices should be aligned with globally accepted standards.
4.	Innovation	The organization should invest in innovation of its products and services, and work across the value chain. If necessary, revise the entire operating model.

		Net Positive Principles
5.	The Big Shift	Achieving net positive can rarely be achieved by carrying on business-as-usual. Organizations typically have to make a substantial shift in terms of their approach and outcomes to achieve net positive outcomes.
6.	Transparency	The organization reports on its net positive progress in a transparent, consistent and authentic manner. Where possible, its net positive outcomes should be independently verified. Furthermore, the organization must clearly define its boundaries and scope, and take both positive and negative impacts into consideration. All trade-offs must also be explained explicitly.
7.	Zero tolerance	A net positive approach implies zero tolerance for unacceptable or irreplaceable natural losses, or ill treatment of individuals and/or communities.
8.	Partnerships	In order to generate bigger positive impacts, the organization should enter into, and leverage, the prowess of wider partnerships and networks.
9.	Throughput	The organization leverages every opportunity for delivering positive impacts across value chains, sectors, systems, and throughput to the natural world and society.
10.	Influence	The organization publicly engages in advocating and influencing policy for positive change.
11.	Inclusive	The organization adopts an inclusive approach at every opportunity, and ensures that the affected communities are involved in the process of creating positive social and environmental impacts.
12.	Restorative	If the key material areas are ecological in nature, the organization must ensure that it applies robust environmentally restorative and socially inclusive methods.

Source: The Net Positive Principles. Forum for the Future. ht t ps:// HYPERLINK http://www/ www. forumforthefuture.org/blog/net-positive-principles. 2016.

Organizations that have embarked on their net positive journeys have gathered critical insights about what works and what does not. These learnings can be categorized as a series of characteristics that every net positive initiative must feature to maximize its chances of succeeding.

1. Making an impact in key areas

The first of these principles revolves around the importance of organizations looking at areas where the greatest potential for impact exists. Naturally, this differs from organization to organization. In the case of IKEA, this potential existed in energy consumption – both energy used in its direct operations and energy used by its customers. On the other hand, for Crown Estate, this equates to influencing the activities of those who occupy the vast tracks of land that the Company owns[157].

2. Changing organizational approach and customs

In order to achieve net positive outcomes, an organization has to change its approach and organizational customs. Business-as-usual is unlikely to achieve any real outcomes, and more radical change in culture and vision is needed. Coca-Cola enterprises, for example, has established joint venture businesses in France, the US, and the UK to transform the PET recycling infrastructure[158]. While this involved capital expenditure that was not directly manufacturing any of its product offerings, it enabled the Company to recycle more packaging than it uses, thus adding value to the environment[159].

3. Collaborating with other organizations

Partnering with other like-minded organizations and companies that have also embraced the net positive approach is likely to yield positive results. As organizations and companies enter into these wider networks, they can learn from each other's experiences, identify best practices, and adopt newer strategies to achieve greater net positive impacts. Kingfisher, for example, collaborates with a number of organizations involving rival businesses, NGOs and suppliers. In 2014,

Kingfisher initiated a new collaborative project called VIA (Verification Impact Analysis) with FSC, IKEA, Tetra Pak and ISEAL. The main objective of the project was establishing a credible methodology for measuring the impact of FSC certification that shows consumers that the Company operates in an environmentally, economically and socially responsible way[160]. In addition, Kingfisher has also worked with the Ellen MacArthur Foundation and Bioregional to develop a 'closed loop calculator', that identifies which products have closed loop credentials (i.e. products made from recycled or renewable materials and employ only renewable energy in their manufacture and use)[161].

4. Expanding the circle of impact

Every opportunity to deliver net positive impacts across the value chains and entire sectors must be leveraged to maximize impact. The impact of all stakeholders and customers must be considered, and potential impact areas must be identified. Companies should then work with each stakeholder to amplify impact across the value chain. BT's Net Good strategy, for example, aims to help customers reduce carbon emissions through its products and services by at least three times (as measured by the end-to-end carbon impact of its business). The mechanisms for expanding their circle of impact includes flexible working services to reduce building needs, efficient transport and mobility, tele-conferencing and reduced travel, and broadband services and dematerialization[162].

Moreover, while businesses aspiring to be net positive may have specific material impact areas they focus on, they must not limit themselves to these areas. They must consider the overall social, economic, and environmental impact of their activities, and exhibit best practice in corporate social responsibility across the spectrum.

5. Policy Influence

Government policies and decisions exert considerable influence on the activities a business undertakes. However, businesses also have the power to influence policy decisions, and are therefore critical levers of societal change[163]. They must use this power to advocate for policies and regulations that enable net positive initiatives. This is not limited to big business as smaller companies can form partnerships and become part of networks to initiate dialogue around policy change that supports net positive.

6. Investing in Net Positive

Businesses integrating net positive in their sustainability goals must invest in the development of products and processes that are environmentally friendly. In some cases, this can imply changing the entire business and revenue models to ensure greater alignment with the net positive strategy. Kingfisher, for example, experimented with an alternative business model such as product hire and repair and the sharing economy, which encourage a continuous reuse of products. Similarly, responding to the shoppers' concern about the environmental impact of disposing of furniture, IKEA tested the solution of renting out furniture instead of selling. Moving from encouraging "mass consumerism" to "mass circularity" marks a radical shift in IKEA's business model[164].

7. Developing a Strong Sustainability Strategy

The sustainability strategy typically forms the basis of a company's net positive approach. A solid and focused sustainability strategy helps businesses in various ways such as improved reputation, cost reduction and engaged staff. A net positive approach magnifies these benefits, and enables companies to secure the supply of resources they rely on, thereby creating a restorative economy[165]. In addition, these businesses can achieve greater operating efficiencies through innovations in product development processes. However, all of this is only possible if net positive ambitions are backed by a sustainability strategy that places equal importance to economic, as well as environmental and social good.

What can be measured can be managed

Once a company has decided to integrate Net Positive into its corporate strategy, it will need to start measuring and managing its Net Positive approach. While doing this, a company is likely to encounter areas that are subjective and where the results are dependent on the approach that the Company adopts in achieving these outcomes.

To ensure that the measurement process is consistent and objective, many lessons have been learnt from practical experience, and are outlined below. Professionals would advise that an organization should comply with seven key measurement principles:

1. Transparency

In order to measure Net Positive, a company is required to undertake a number of calculations and approximations, using multiple data sources. Naturally, many assumptions have to be made to conduct these calculations. While rules and standards cannot be developed for every eventuality, it is important that the organization is transparent about the methodology it applies to calculate its social and environmental impact, so that results can be compared and contrasted by other organizations/individuals.

In 2013, BT, which is a UK-based broadband company, launched its Net Good programme, which aimed to deliver a net positive environmental impact. BT regularly evaluates its positive and negative impacts, and publishes a detailed methodology used to measure impact. Through the provision of bandwidth, BT enables workers to work remotely using a broadband connection, eliminating the need to commute or travel for work. This reduces carbon emissions, as well as energy use within the office environment. Rebound effects of increased energy use in the telecommuter's home are also taken into consideration. BT's approach, methodology, assumptions and data sources are publically available and published online.

2. Consistency

Organizations should evaluate the positive and negative impacts in a consistent manner and across the value chain. This will allow the business to analyze the net environmental or social impact of a product or service. To illustrate, if a product's positive carbon footprint (e.g. carbon saved by using a product) is being assessed, it is imperative to also take into account the negative carbon footprint that emerged from the product's manufacturing.

3. Completeness

Economic, social and environmental impacts should be measured completely and accurately. In the eventuality that information for a material area is not available, companies should use a conservative estimate rather than omitting or leaving a gap. However, in such an eventuality, the assumptions have to be clarified and the intentions for acquiring the data should be specified by the company.

To illustrate, TUI Group, a tourism business, partnered with PwC and the Travel Foundation to measure the impact of 60,000 TUI customers who visited 8 hotels in Cyprus during 2013. The methodology used for this exercise was PwC's 'Total Impact Measurement & Management" (TIMM) methodology. The study measured and valued a wide range of economic, fiscal, social and environmental impacts. This was a pioneering initiative, as it was the first time the methodology had been applied to tourism. The impact assessment was the most comprehensive assessment ever undertaken for tourism operation within a holiday destination. The positive economic and tax benefits constituted the greatest impact – amounting to €84 per guest per night. The positive impact was far greater than the negative environmental (-€4) and social (-€0.2) costs. However, it was announced that the exercise provided a one-year (2013) snapshot and excluded the impact of the construction of the hotels[166].

4. Separation of different categories of impacts

Since trading off or balancing impacts (e.g. social and carbon) against each other is a difficult task, companies should compare these impacts at the project level, but keep them separate. For example, the positive impact of reducing water usage cannot be compared to the negative impact of poor working conditions for employees. Similar to the different categories of impacts, positive and negative impacts also have to be separated. Positive impacts of a particular project or product do not necessarily compensate for negative impacts. Therefore, these two types of impacts should be disclosed separately while comparing them at an individual project level.

5. Leveraging existing approaches

While the concept of net positive is relatively new, there are nevertheless some existing methods such as the Greenhouse Gas Protocol, and Life Cycle Assessments (LCA) and Product Carbon Footprints (PCF), which feature tried and tested means of assessing positive carbon impacts. LCA systematically assesses multiple environmental impacts of a product, activity or a process over the life cycle of that product, activity or process. This methodology involves an end-to-end analysis of the product or service that the company is providing, and covers all raw materials, production processes, transportation, usage and disposal of the product. Another methodology to analyze carbon impact is the Carbon Footprint Analysis, referred as Greenhouse Gas Emissions Assessment, which evaluates the greenhouse gas emissions by the production of a product or any given activity that contributes to global warming. In the first stage of analysis, the emissions of carbon, sulfur hexafluoride, and methane are assessed. After the emissions are found, the assessment converts the output into carbon dioxide equivalents ($CO2e$)[167].

6. Data Sharing

It is critical for businesses to ensure that they are transparent about the boundaries and assumptions they use for data collection. It is equally important for companies to share the data that is collected. This will not only mainstream the Net Positive discourse within the company, but also enable companies to learn from each other's best practices. This is particularly applicable for companies which are at similar stages within a supply chain, as their measurement of carbon footprint (both negative and positive) and resource use will require similar metrics and indicators. Data sharing in the Net Positive agenda brings the issue of impacts in the limelight and encourages other players in the industry to follow suit and start measuring their impact.

For example, in a bold move, Tesco started publishing food waste data in 2013. While the announcement created ripples in the media and led to public outcry, Tesco understood that it was something that needed to trigger a debate about a pressing global challenge. The company revealed that Tesco stores and distribution centres wasted 28,500 tonnes of food in the first six months of 2013. Tesco paved a pathway for other food retailers to start measuring and capturing the impact of food wastage, and some of UK's biggest grocers vowed to follow Tesco's lead[168].

7. Net Positive journey dashboard

These dashboards present information about the performance of Net Positive aspiring companies in each impact area, and across their lines of business and/or the range of companies within the larger corporate group. Companies like Kingfisher use such dashboards to present the operating company performance summary, and scores each company within the group in each of the relevant impact areas (e.g. natural resource usage, employees, community development, etc.) to demonstrate progress.

Making it happen: the roadmap to Net Positive

With regard to actual management activities, i.e. the steps that must be taken to start implementing a Net Positive strategy, the Forum of the Future and The Climate Group published a series of management steps that can be taken to ensure that the development of Net Positive within an organization is a consistent and objective process. This section summarizes and outlines these considerations.

Materiality

Materiality refers to the significance of an area or impact that an organization has on its internal and external stakeholders, as well as environment and society at large. For example, a natural resource such as wood or timber would be a material impact area for a company manufacturing wooden furniture. Furthermore, a material impact area could also be a space in which the company can make a transformational change. Consequently, materiality helps organizations decide which areas they should measure and focus their efforts on viz-a-vis Net Positive and environmental sustainability.

However, an organization has to assess the entire supply chain and beyond to identify material impacts. They have to evaluate the material impact along its value chain and the impact it has beyond its own boundaries. For example, customers and suppliers of a company have their own sets of impacts, which have to be evaluated. In a similar vein, to get a holistic picture of material impacts, a company has to consider its entire product range and its operations to identify material impact areas. Thus, companies looking to become Net Positive have to adopt an approach that is suited to the strategy and risks associated with their businesses. Furthermore, this approach has to be reviewed regularly to ensure that the material impacts identified are relevant, and if any new material impact areas have to be added. With regard to disclosure, companies need to be transparent about how material impact areas were identified, the areas in which the organization has been selective, and where the boundaries were drawn.

Determining Materiality: Kingfisher's Case[169]

Kingfisher is Europe's leading home improvement retailer, operating nearly 1200 stores and growing omni-channel operations across 10 countries in Europe. Kingfisher's sales in the year ended 31 January 2017 were over US$ 14.7 billion across the multiple brands it operates. The company launched its Net Positive commitment in 2012, with targets in various areas including sustainable home products, energy efficiency and responsible sourcing of wood and paper. Today, a quarter of Kingfisher's sales are from products that improve the sustainability of people's homes[170].

In order to establish materiality, Kingfisher takes into account a wide range of social, environmental and economic issues that are relevant to its business and stakeholders. Prioritization of issues is conducted through extensive consultation with internal and external stakeholders. Issues that are of foremost importance to these stakeholders and have a considerable impact on Kingfisher's business are identified, keeping in view the commercial, operational and reputational risks and opportunities. The continual engagement has enabled the company to streamline Net Positive aspirations and targets, and is based on the following process:

1. Internal Review: Kingfisher conducts a stakeholder mapping exercise which helps identify priority stakeholders that the company needs to engage with in order to pursue its Net Positive goals. Moreover, this exercise allows Kingfisher to collate and review feedback and information from internal and external sources.

2. External Review: Kingfisher regularly engages directly with stakeholders through different means including face-to-face meetings and investor roadshows. Furthermore, it also has membership of organizations including Forum for the Future, BSR and the Ellen MacArthur Foundation. By means of a combined review with all these external stakeholders, Kingfisher is able to identify a list of issues which are most material to its stakeholders.

3. Prioritization: Kingfisher works with external stakeholders through workshops and specialist forums, and with internal stakeholders through Net Positive Network meetings to prioritize areas for action and review processes.

Measuring Impact

To evaluate the extent of impact that an organization has, it is important to assess the extent and aspects in which the existing system has changed. Important areas for consideration are:

1. *The innovation*

The company develops a product that has the potential for bringing about a Net Positive change in a material impact area.

2. *The baseline*

The company must identify the baseline against which impact is being compared, and this baseline must be reviewed and altered (if necessary) periodically. Companies typically choose to compare with the market average performance, and/or to compare with the specific materials used before the product was developed.

3. *Displacement and rebound*

In this regard, the company has to consider if its product or innovation has a rebound effect, i.e., has it shifted the material impact in another direction, or if the material impact is in fact Net Positive. Moreover, a business must also consider if its innovation encourages the customer to cause negative impact. For example, an innovation that enables an automotive manufacturer to save fuel and reduce carbon footprint can also stimulate a rebound effect as it can encourage customers to drive more.

4. *Timeline and attribution of benefits*

In some special circumstances, as the innovation ages, the extent of impact tends to diminish, and the attribution to the business is lower. Companies need to account for this, especially if the decline in impact is sharp.

5. Responsibility for the change

The extent of a business's responsibility for the positive impact has to be established when measuring Net Positive. Companies typically use two methods:

(i) All or Nothing, which maintains that no positive gain would have been established had it not been for the company's innovation, or
(ii) Proportional, which involves the assignment of responsibility to different parties along the supply chain (e.g. an actual manufacturer of the innovation).

Companies need to address each of these areas, and disclose the methodology they have employed in doing so.

Extrapolation

To measure Net Positive, businesses often need assumptions and extrapolations to capture and quantify the impacts across the entire organization. For example, as part of its Net Positive strategy, a company may sell products which allow the reduction of carbon or water footprint. However, the actual amount of carbon emissions or water wastage avoided will depend on the customer's usage and circumstances.

Therefore, the business must make and disclose reasonable assumptions based on research and data. In addition, a sample of the representative population where the company is operating also has to be calculated, as water and carbon footprint varies significantly from place to place. While industry averages can also be used, caution has to be exercised as they are less accurate than targeted surveys and studies. The sources of data and information for the assumptions, and the actual extrapolations also have to be disclosed.

Measuring Outcomes

There are several ways in which a business can create positive and negative value. The most obvious and direct way a business can create positive value is through products and services that enable customers to reduce their carbon or water footprint. Furthermore, businesses can enable others to create positive impact by partnering with them or encouraging them. In some cases, the domino effect of this contribution can be significantly greater than the value created directly by offering products and services. Therefore, the question that arises is: How much of an impact can a business claim?

In this regard, businesses must address the following concerns in this area:

1. If a company's product or service offerings help customers reduce their carbon or water footprints, how can this reduction in footprint be calculated?
2. If a company enables another organization to create value, how can the value enabled be calculated?
3. In each of the above scenarios, there are multiple factors which determine the creation of value. How much of that value creation can the company claim?

Very often businesses offer products/services, and also encourage other organizations downstream to create positive value. In such a scenario, businesses must be careful to avoid double counting. While there is no generally accepted best practice in this area, businesses must be transparent and disclose footprint avoided and value created separately. In a similar vein, disclosure of the calculations and assumptions for each of these impacts is also recommended.

Assurance

A company with a Net Positive commitment must ensure that the information it is collecting and using is accurate. Assurance practices must be put into place to gain confidence in the data. However, these practices must be rolled out gradually, and rigorous assurance practices involving external experts should not be integrated at the onset of the Net Positive initiative to avoid wasting resource. Assurance should be brought in after a sufficient time has passed allowing for the learning curve effect to take place.

Transparency

Net Positive businesses must be transparent about every aspect of business that influences the Net Positive impact areas. This can be achieved by making the information publicly available, or through direct engagement with the different stakeholders. Transparency will enable stakeholders to trust the business, and also provide important insights. At minimum, a company embarking on its Net Positive journey must disclose its aims and ambitions for Net Positive, and report its achievements on a regular basis. The calculations, methodologies, sources of information, and assumptions should also be disclosed.

Measuring Impact Areas: the Net Positive bottom line

Companies choose their material impact areas based on the nature of their business operations, and product and service offerings. In the Net Positive realm, typically companies have focused their efforts on five main areas, namely carbon, water, social, resource use, and ecological impact. While the methodologies for measurement may vary from one area to another, transparency and disclosure of methods and calculations have to be ensured across the board.

Carbon

In the carbon domain, companies aim to remove or avoid generating more carbon than they create at any point in the value chain. Kilogram is the standard metric to measure the carbon footprint, and there are well established guidelines and standards that organizations can use to measure their carbon impact. To begin with, Net Positive companies should measure the carbon created and avoided separately across the supply chain. Greenhouse Gas Protocol Scopes can be used, as they distinguish between upstream, operations and downstream impacts generated. More advanced measurements of carbon employ distinctive geographic and product analysis to measure total carbon impact.

Water

Companies looking to become Net Positive in water must focus on two areas, namely access and quality. They should aim to create greater access to water and better quality water than they consume across their value chain. However, the quantity of water consumed is a relative concept, as a certain amount of water consumed in a water-scarce area has much higher significance than the same amount of water consumed in a water-poor area. In terms of quality, water can be classified as Blue (fresh surface water and ground water), Green (rain water that stays on the land) and Grey (an indicator of fresh water pollution). Consumption can be measured in liters, gallons or cubic meters, but a consistent metric should be used across the value chain. Similar to carbon, impact has to be measured separately, with a clear distinction between footprint avoided and value created. However, water's quality dimension has to be taken into consideration and the distinction between footprint created and avoided between Green, Blue and Grey water has to be made. This is particularly important for companies that are involved with the agricultural sector, where the distinction between blue and green water has to be made clearly. Geographic and product analysis can be measured separately for more advanced measurements of water footprint. Tools are also available to facilitate companies to understand if they are operating in water-stressed or water-rich areas. However, good practice is yet to be established in location-specific analyses across a company's supply chain.

Social Impact

Being Net Positive in terms of social impact implies that a company's business operations across the supply chain do not destroy social value, and in fact contribute towards the creation of social and human capital. While human capital comprises of people's skill sets, capacities, and motivation, social capital focuses on institutions that enable the development and maintenance of human capital, in partnership with other dimensions of capital such as communities, schools, voluntary associations, etc. Thus, a Net Positive commitment in social capital would involve the enabling of conditions which create more social and human capital across the supply chain. In the upstream segment supply chain, companies can focus on the way they handle suppliers and their employees. In operations, Net Positive can be created by emphasizing working conditions, opportunities for professional development for company employees, and the impact of the company's operations on the local community. Finally, focusing on customers' use of the company's products and services, and what these products enable the customers to do can generate Net Positive in the social domain. Measuring social value is a challenging task, as there are many components of social value, each with its own metric, thus making aggregation and comparison a difficult task. As a result, the social value in each segment of the business and operations must be segregated, and indicators for each segment must be developed. The company must also determine a way to aggregate the information to present a realistic and accurate estimate of social value created. The methodology and calculations must be disclosed to ensure transparency.

Measuring Social Impact: The Crown Estate's Total Contribution Methodology[171]

In 2013, The Crown Estate, one of the largest property managers in the United Kingdom, introduced a new methodology for reporting on sustainable business. This new methodology, titled Total Contribution, demonstrates the wider impacts that the company activities have on each category of capitals on which they depend. The activities are split into three categories:

1. Direct activity: carried out by the company
2. Indirect activity: commissioned by the company but carried out by the supply chain
3. Enabled activity: carried out by customers on the company's land

The Total Contribution approach considers the company's impact in the following areas:

- Financial resources: Economic resources which allow the company to run and grow its business
- Physical resources: Property, plant and equipment, and other manufactured goods the company uses
- Natural resources: Resources supplied by the ecosystem (e.g. minerals, carbon sequestration and biodiversity provided by the natural environment)
- People: The skills, competencies and experience of employees
- Know-how: Collective expertise and processes
- Networks: Relationships and trust between stakeholders including customers, communities and business partners

Since the array of impacts is so diverse, the methodology uses economic valuation as a common unit of measurement for all the indicators. If the data lends itself to a financial measurement (e.g. amount spent on employees' healthcare), the calculation is fairly simple. For data which is presented as a non-financial unit of measurement (e.g. carbon emission), the appropriate social cost/benefit value unit is researched and identified to be used in the economic valuation. For direct impacts, this calculation is a straight forward task. However, for indirect impacts where data is not easily available, assumptions and estimations have to be applied. 60 performance indicators, which reflect both positive and negative impacts, have been developed to cover direct, indirect and enabled impacts. An economic value is ascribed to each indicator, and the positive/negative value for each capital is calculated to obtain the net value. Each capital-specific net value is added or subtracted to or from the gross-value-added (financial resources).

Material Use

The material that businesses use can come from renewable or non-renewable sources, but the focus here will be on renewable resources, particularly non- energy resources. The consumption or use of this material impacts the sustainability of the resource. Being Net Positive in material use implies that the business renews more resources than it consumes across the value chain. In addition, businesses aiming to be Net Positive in material use must source these materials in a responsible manner.

With regard to measurement, a different unit is associated with each resource. Organizations that use a natural resource like wood will use the number of trees they use as a unit of measurement. While this may not be a specific measure, it is a sufficient one, as it paves the way forward for establishing how Net Positive can be achieved (planting more trees, in this case). However, what is also important to note is the sustainability in sourcing the resources, and the entire value chain has to be assessed to confirm that the resources are coming from a sustainable source. This is critical for ensuring that the resource will continue to be available in the future. Reduction of waste generation is also an area that organizations should pay attention to, and efforts must be undertaken to derive positive value from waste (e.g. creation of energy through waste).

The factors that organizations need to consider and establish good practice in pertain to the quality and offsetting of resources. A comparison between resources used (quality of old trees) and resources added (quality and type of new trees planted) has to be conducted to create Net Positive value in a meaningful way. Moreover, the conditions under which offsetting can be claimed also have to be established and agreed upon. Businesses must also be careful in separating the footprint created and avoided and the value created in each resource or material used. This strategy is to be applied across the supply chain. For a more advanced measure, the geographic and product analysis should be undertaken separately, and the information should be aggregated in a systematic and transparent manner.

Ecological

In producing goods and services, businesses use and impact the natural ecosystems such as soil, land, biodiversity and geological resources. Thus, being a Net Positive business implies that the organization enhances or restores natural capital more than it consumes. Since natural capital is comprised of various elements, the measurement for each element is different. This makes measurement and aggregation difficult. Nevertheless, organizations should apply similar principles in the measurement of ecological impact as all other impact areas. Therefore, footprint created, avoided, and value created should be measured separately across the supply chain. Similarly, advanced measurements should involve a geographic and product analysis, and a comparison of the quality of the natural capital consumed and created should be undertaken.

Critical Success Factors

As organizations develop their Net Positive strategies and put initiatives into place to spur implementation, there are certain critical success factors that have to be in place. These factors will ensure that the net positive impact that the business organization is both meaningful and long-lasting. In planning and practically making its transition towards a net positive business, Majid Al Futtaim has learned a number of lessons that can provide a platform for other organizations to follow suit. Some of these are new and unique, while others confirm and stress the points mentioned in this chapter. The list below is an attempt to distill these critical success factors, with the aim of these becoming guiding notes for any company joining this movement.

1. Materiality: focus on areas that matter

An organization aiming to become Net Positive must understand where its biggest impacts are - the ones that substantially affect the business's ability to deliver value. These are the areas where attention should be focused. Conducting a robust materiality review before setting off is vital for the success of any Net Positive strategy. This will help show the organization where to direct its efforts according to the nature and type of business and its products and services (e.g. a property company should focus on its buildings). The organization should use valuable resource and time to focus on the areas that really matter and where the business can make the most difference.

2. Initial Business Case: Management buy-in is key

Net Positive delivers business as well as social and environmental benefits. However, the feasibility of adopting a Net Positive approach should be well scrutinized to ensure it's the right approach for the company at that point in time. This is critical to achieve business buy-in, at all levels, and to move away from the "nice to have" category. Buy-in needs to come from the top to secure budget and support but ultimately net positive needs to be embedded across the business to ensure a lasting impact and quick and effective progress.

3. Boundaries: think big but know your limits

To achieve Net Positive, it is important for a business to set meaningful boundaries: the impact a business has affects its staff, customers and suppliers. It is not feasible for a company to tackle everything. A clear line needs to be drawn, but it is vital to achieve the right balance. The Net Positive strategy must refrain from being too narrow in its focus, as this implies that the business would miss out on potentially high influence areas. At the same time, the focus must not be too wide or expansive, as this can result in the organizational resources being spread too thinly.

4. Footprint: measure, measure, measure

Calculation of a business's footprint can be a laborious effort, but it is an activity that is integral for goal-setting. A business must know what its impacts are so it can effectively target the hot spots for priority action. Time, resources and budgets must be invested wisely, and determining the footprint is vital to this decision. Not knowing its footprint comes at the high risk of leading financial and human resources down a long and ineffective path to Net Positive.

5. Strong Foundation: net positive as a core business process

Organizations should invest time in building their network and resources across the business. A robust internal governance structure needs to be developed to ensure that progress is not hinged on a few people within the organization. Human resources that have a strong background in environmental sustainability and corporate performance must be engaged. Capacity building must be undertaken to enable employees to steer the organization towards its Net Positive goals. A strong reporting process must also be established for this governance structure and human resources to work in an effective manner.

6. Transparency: the age of open data

Being Net Positive is an ambitious commitment for any organization to make. While all the factors outlined above are critical for a Net Positive commitment to be realized, it is equally important that the organization is held accountable against its commitment. Since the timelines for Net Positive can span over decades, it is easy to lose track of progress. By publishing its targets and methodology, and reporting against every year, an organization can streamline its efforts and be confident in its claims and commitment.

7. Collaboration: a stakeholder approach

Net Positive is an emerging area within corporate sustainability. The scale of the challenge implies that no business can do it without collaborating with and learning from others. The spectrum of organizations that can assist each other is wide and includes knowledge partners, customers, as well as companies with established track record of Net Positive delivery. These could be external to the committing business, or related to it (across the supply chain).

The Future is Net Positive

Businesses around the world are adopting strategies that incorporate sustainability into mainstream corporate value creation approaches. Net positive is one path to sustainable value creation. While best practices and guidelines on measurement and reporting in the area are still developing, companies around the world are driving strategic change to integrate Net Positive into their sustainability commitments. Companies are increasingly realizing why sustainability is material to their business, and why it is imperative to take urgent action [172]. The motivation for embedding Net Positive into their sustainability strategies is diverse. Several organizations are driven towards Net Positive to keep abreast with competitors, while others are motivated by corporate responsibility and branding concerns [173].

The scope for large scale change driven through corporate sustainability efforts is also expanding as the fourth industrial revolution unravels unprecedented possibilities for innovation and new breakthroughs. This naturally has a dramatic impact on business via supply and demand routes. The disruption in the production process presents an opportunity for businesses to explore new ways of serving existing needs. On the other hand, the prevalence of big data implies that consumers are more aware and engaged, resulting in a change in the nature, design, and type of goods and services demanded [174]. This change in the demand and supply landscape is forcing companies to modify the way they do business, and achieve profitability and sustainability targets.

No matter why they do it, and how, more and more companies are now convinced that Net Positive is part of their future.

(Endnotes)

157 Eig ht steps to ma ke t he idea of 'net posit ive' more t ha n simply jargon. The Guardian. https://w w w.theguardian.com/ sustainable-business/ eight-steps-net-positive-jargon-business. April 2014.
158 Ibid.
159 Our Approach to Sustainable Packaging. The Coca Cola Company. HYPERLINK http://www.coca-colacompany.com/stories/our-approach-t http://w w w.coca-colacompany.com/stories/our-approach-t o-sustainable-packaging
160 Kingfisher Net Positive Report 2014-2015. Kingfisher. 2015
161 Kingfisher takes commercial 'make do and mend ' into the mainstream. The Guardian. https://w w w.t heg uardian.com/ sustainable-business/ sustainability-case-studies-kingfisher-ellen-macarthur-foundation-circular-economy. May 2014
162 Net Good: Pathway to Carbon Net Positive.
163 Why influencing public policy has never been more important for business. Forum for the Future. https://www.forumforthefu- ture.org/blog/wh y-influencing-public-policy-has-never-been-m ore-important-business. 2015.
164 Ikea tests renting out furniture as eco-friendly plan. The Telegraph. ht t ps://w w w.teleg raph.co.u k / busi ness/2018/01/24/i kea-test s-renting-furniture-eco-friendly-plan/. January 2018.
165 Eig ht steps to ma ke t he idea of 'net posit ive' more t ha n simply jargon. The Guardian. https://w w w.theguardian.com/ sustainable-business/ eight-steps-net-positive-jargon-business. April 2014.
166 Measuring Your Way to Net Positive. Forum for the Future & The Climate Group. 2016
167 Similarities and Differences between Carbon Footprint and Life Cycle Analysis. The Balance. https://w ww.thebalance.com/carbo n-footprint-vs-life-cycle-2 878059. November 2016
168 Tesco sparked debate on food waste. The Guardian. https:// HYPERLINK http://www/ www. theguardian.com/sustainable-business/ sustainability-case-studie s-tesco-waste. May 2014.

169 Net Positive Report 2014/15: Delivering our strategy sustain- ably. Kingfisher. https:// HYPERLINK http://www.kingfisher.com/sustainability/files/ www.kingfisher.com/sustainability/files/ reports/cr report 2015/2015 Net Positive Report.pdf

170 Sustainability Report 2016/2017. Kingfisher. https://www.king-fisher.com/sustainability/files/reports/cr report 2017/index.html

171 Total Contribution Methodology. The Crown Estate. https:// w w w.t hecrow nestate.co.u k /media/1023089/t he-crown-estat e-methodology-2 017.pdf. 2017

172 Corporate Sustainability at a Crossroads. David Kiron, Nina Kruschwitz, Martin Reeves, Holger Rubel, Alexander Meyer Zum Felde. HYPERLINK http://sloanreview.mit.edu/projects/corporate-sustainabilit http://sloanreview.mit.edu/projects/corporate-sustainabilit y-at-a-crossroads/#chapter-2. May 23, 2013.

173 Joining Forces: Collaboration and Leadership for Sustainability. David Kiron, Nina Kruschwitz, Knut Haanaes, Martin Reeves, Sonja-Katrin Fuisz-Kehrbach, George Kell. HYPERLINK http://sloanreview/ http://sloanreview.mit.edu. Jan. 12, 2015.

174 The Fourth Industrial Revolution: what it means, how to respond. Klaus Schwab. https://w w w.weforum.org/agenda/2016/01/th e-fou rth-i ndust r ia l-revolut ion-what-it-mea ns-a nd-how-to- respond/. 14 Jan, 2016.

Chapter 5

Sustainability in the age of the Fourth Industrial Revolution

The age of the fourth industrial revolution

As technology changes the shape and form of all human interaction, it is also fueling a revolutionary change within all industries. All aspects of production, consumption and logistics are already undergoing rapid and revolutionary change, thus spurring what is commonly referred to as the Fourth Industrial Revolution (4IR). While change in the first industrial revolution stemmed from the introduction of mechanization of production, the second and the third revolutions were a result of new technologies such as electricity, telephones, and computers. The advent of digital computers in the 1950s paved way for mass production that was enabled by automation. The next phase that came with the rise of digital communication catalyzed an information revolution which connected the world through networks such as the internet and mobile technologies[175].

In this landscape, the impact of the fourth industrial revolution on industry is already transformational, and we are still at the beginning. While the most obvious impact today of the 4IR has the manufacturing sector (with 3D printing, robotics, machine learning, etc.), its potential extends across all sectors. One key element of the 4IR is the Internet of Things, which refers to the use of "intelligently connected devices and systems to leverage data gathered through embedded sensors and actuators in machines and other physical objects"[176]. In simple terms, the IoT is essentially a system where items in the physical world, and sensors within or attached to these items, are connected to the Internet through wireless and wired Internet connections.[177] The societal, cultural and business impact of this is large, and is only expected to increase over time. Estimates suggest that by 2020 there will be over 26 billion connected devices[178].

The collective impact of the IoT, encompassed with a wider range of technologies such as big data analytics, artificial intelligence, robotics, augmented and virtual reality, blockchain, will be considerable and visible. These technologies will extend beyond simple communication to the realms of connecting inanimate and living things, and generate data on daily interactions. Today, wearable digital sensory health devices (such as FitBit) can generate data and create a connected ecosystem of human activity. While a simple device, the implications of future version of this "health-sensor" connectivity are enormous. Sensors will be leveraged to collect data from all aspects of our daily lives (health, education, shopping, location, etc.). The physical objects being connected will possess sensors, each of which can monitor a particular condition, and the IoT enables these sensors to get connected to each other, and generate frequent data feeds that can collectively provide useful information to a company's systems and employees. Machine-to-machine communications are also a facet of IoT that will reduce dependence on central cloud-based applications. This, in turn, will allow for greater automation of basic and recurring tasks[179].

This bloc of technologies creates cyber-physical systems that fuse advanced digital technology and artificial intelligence with people and machines. IoT creates new data sources and the frequency of this exercise generates large quantities of information. Robotics and augmented reality technology is facilitating greater automation of manufacturing processes and generating more data. This data can be mined using analytics, thus creating more intelligence and insights into products, preferences and processes. Moreover, technologies such as drones, cloud computing, and 3D printing further push the innovation and production frontier for all businesses, irrespective of size. In fact, small and medium enterprises, particularly start-ups, are now spearheading tech-based product and productivity innovations[180].

The impact of these technologies is multi-faceted and far-reaching. Innovative businesses are leveraging augmented reality to design products that alter human experience. In health, for example, companies like AccuVein are using Augmented Reality (AR) technology to reduce patient discomfort during the process of drawing blood or injecting intravenous (IV) medicines and fluids. Research shows that 40% of IVs miss the vein on the first stick, with the numbers getting worse for children and the elderly. AccuVein has designed a hand-held scanner that allows for better vein visualization. The scanner projects the vasculature map over the patient's skin and shows nurses and doctors where veins are in the patients' bodies.[181]

In the health sector, another innovation using in early 2018 Uber introduced a new service called Uber Health to provide reliable and comfortable transportation to patients. The new business line aims to provide a ride-hailing platform that can be used by healthcare providers to book rides for their patients through a centralized web-based dashboard, eliminating the need for the patients to have the Uber app themselves.[182]

In the tourism industry, virtual reality enables companies to give consumers a virtual trial in the form of guided tours using VR gear. It has allowed tourism companies such as Thomas Cook to help their customers virtually trial the experience at various destinations before they purchase a holiday package. Using Samsung's Gear VR, potential vacationers can visit the company's flagship stores in the UK, Belgium and Germany to experience a series of virtual reality holidays by getting a life-like look at a hotel before booking and a virtual experience of holiday excursions in select countries. Thomas Cook's Try Before You Fly program has been a phenomenal success, as the program managed to almost double the number of New York excursions within a year of launching the program.[183]

Industries such as beauty and fashion are employing 3D printing to develop product prototypes. In 2017, Adidas introduced a new trainer featuring a 3D-printed sole.[184] Following suit, Nike, which is one of Adidas's main rival firms, also started developing shoe prototypes from thermoplastic polyurethane (TPU) material. The ultimate aim of this initiative is to reduce the time and cost of manufacturing the product, while also enhancing comfort for consumers.[185]

Business disruption: a new world of opportunities

The 4IR technological advances have immense potential to generate speedy and powerful disruption for businesses. A direct impact is already being felt on product design and the operational processes used to manufacture the product. As manufacturing facilities become more complex but also more agile owing to automation, they will have the ability to support mass customization of products without any delays pertaining to machine downtime. Consequently, businesses will be able to combine the intelligence from the existing products with more streamlined and optimized processes to produce targeted products that can serve different customer segments[186]. This mass customization in production will be in parallel to unprecedented power of data analytics. Big data will drive decisions about products, processes and productivity and will make business intelligence systems more robust and enable better decision-making[187]. They allow businesses to gain competitive advantage, creating new revenue opportunities, and improving the bottom line. Research demonstrates that firms typically apply these analytics to big data to focus cross-selling and up-selling, gain a better understanding of individual customer needs, and optimize pricing[188].

Businesses in every sector are using big data to cut costs and/or increase revenue. In the retail sector, Target, an American retail giant, has been using big data to create a pregnancy detection model to promote sales of baby products. Target assigns a unique consumer ID that tracks a consumer's purchases. This data is documented to develop the customer's purchase history (credit card usage, products purchased every month) and demographic profile (e.g. gender, marital status, number of children, etc). This data, coupled with data from shopper registries for new mothers, enables Target to track shopping habits and trends, and develop a list of 25 products that are regularly purchased by expecting mothers. By applying predictive analysis to this data and shopper history, Target is to identify pregnant women in their second trimester – even those who have not notified Target about their pregnancy. The company uses this information to estimate the delivery date and push certain products (such as cribs, diapers, and milk) and specific promotions for new mothers and babies. Since 2002, when this shopper analysis first began, Target increased its revenue from US$ 44 billion to US$ 67 billion by 2010.[189]

In the automotive industry, companies such as Ford and Tesla are gathering real time data to ultimately develop efficient and safer cars. Ford gathers extensive data on fuel efficiency, safety, quality and emissions through in-car sensors and remote application management software. Real-time analysis of this data allows Ford engineers to identify and resolve issues without any time lag, and also analyze how different cars perform in different weather conditions. Ford is also using big data to monitor driver behavior through in-car sensors such as smart cameras, radars, and sensors. The company uses this data to optimize manufacturing efficiency and driver safety.[190]

Tesla, on the other hand, is taking the usage big data to the next level. Real-time data generated through sensors and smart technology in Tesla cars is used to generate data-intensive maps that track a range of parameters including location hazards and the increase in traffic and speed over a certain segment of a given route. The ultimate aim of gathering this data is to leverage it to develop safer driver-less cars in the future.[191]

In addition to advances in processes and automation of manufacturing facilities and smarter supply chains, these technological advances will also address issues related to energy usage and working environment. Data analytics, robotics and automation, for example, have the potential to maximize the efficiency of energy use and create a safer working environment. In the manufacturing sector, machine vision is one application that has the potential of making the production process considerably safer. Cameras which are several times more sensitive than the human eye enable the development of machine-vision tools, which can identify microscopic defects in products. On a more macro level, factories are leveraging the self-driving robotic technology via collaborative robots or "cobots" that can co-work with humans to make the production process more efficient and safe. Artificial intelligence allows these cobots to take instructions from humans and efficiently perform a task.

Beyond robotics, AI is facilitating manufacturing through algorithms that are pivotal for predictive maintenance for factor equipment. Sensors that track operating conditions and performance of factory equipment generate data that allows companies to forecast the time and nature of potential breakdowns and malfunctions. AI-powered automation of procurement processes, for example, can then order new supplies, identify challenges pertaining to the production line, and minimize energy consumption. It also enables managers to take precise and targeted corrective or preemptive actions to ensure that the production process remains safe and seamless.

While manufacturers have been using predictive analysis and big data for a while, AI has catalyzed this process by accounting for and process a much larger volume of real-time information.[192] Beyond scale, AI also has the advantage of speed and application, as it can process data at an unprecedented pace, resulting into real-time decisions and real-time actions.[193] In terms of energy efficiency, AI presents immense conservation opportunities for companies. From designing energy-efficient products to minimizing the amount of energy used in the production process, AI can assist the next generation of companies in reducing their carbon footprint. Airbus, a leading aircraft manufacturer, is experimenting with generative design to arrive at the lightest possible part for new aircrafts. Lighter parts not only reduce manufacturing costs, but also improve the energy performance of the aircraft. Based on the part's design goal and the specified building materials inputted by the company's engineers, the AI software can generate thousands of creative and commercially feasible iterations of the part. The company can then decide on the optimal solution based on the weight and energy savings each iteration can achieve.[194]

IoT sensors will also further the environmental sustainability agenda, as they allow for better and faster detection of environmental pollution. IBM is investing in developing cloud-connected IoT sensors which will monitor the natural gas infrastructure. Using this technology, oil and gas companies will be able to track their facilities and identify leaks in real-time, thus reducing pollution and waste, and preventing catastrophic events such caused by chemical and methane leaks.[195]

However, the impact of 4IR will not be limited to product and service design. Whole supply chains, as well as transportation and logistics services, will witness a huge impact in terms of efficiency and productivity improvements. The application of artificial intelligence will minimize material waste and reduce the incidence of delays in production and delivery. Automation will enable manufacturers to be connected with upstream and downstream stakeholders, as well as customers. Through the use of sensors, tags and other devices, IoT and visualization technologies will allow better and real-time tracking of assets, as well as inventory and components. In 2015, Cisco and DHL estimated that US$ 1.9 trillion of fiscal savings could be generated in the global supply chain and logistics sector through the use of IoT devices and asset tracking tech solutions[196].

Finally, technology will also have an impact on the jobs and employment landscape. As digitization and automation continue, the workplace will undergo a seismic change. While there are different estimates of the extent to which jobs may become automated, change is nevertheless inevitable[197]. Labor-saving technology and automation have already reduced jobs in the manufacturing sector, and this trend can be seen spreading to other sectors, including the service industry. The issue of job losses owing to technology and automation is particularly problematic for developing countries that typically rely on the availability of cheap labor as an economic incentive for investment from emerging and developed markets.

The labor market will also witness a shift in the kind of skill sets demanded. This can potentially result in rising inequality, as the market for middle-skilled workers are most susceptible to "technological unemployment"[198]. Nevertheless, automation will also create jobs in the face of new business processes and skill sets demanded. The potential impact of automation has to be analyzed with regard to individual activities and skills, not entire occupations. Automation impacts each activity within the value chain in a different manner, and less then 5% of occupations are likely to be automated completely. However, even partial automation is likely to have a far-reaching impact on employment and earnings[199].

Sustainability in the age of the Fourth Industrial Revolution

As the frontiers of innovation expand, a range of new production techniques that spur creative destruction are becoming available to businesses. In the specific context of environmental sustainability, green innovations are generating large and often untapped strategic advantage for businesses. Breakthrough technologies can be harnessed to create low-carbon solutions and reduce emissions. Moreover, renewable sources of energy have the potential to drive innovation and generate competitive advantage that did not previously exist.

Most importantly, the business imperative to invest in sustained innovation around 4IR technologies stems from the potential of these innovations to expand market opportunities. They enable businesses to produce and sell more while achieving cost reductions, exploring new revenue streams and securing the planet's future [200]. Therefore, it is critical for businesses to explore certain influential action areas that have the potential to make the fourth industrial revolution a sustainable one.

Clean Energy

The global power sector accounts for 25% of global greenhouse gas emissions[201]. Coal, which generates air and water pollution, is the most commonly used source (circa 41%) for electricity generation today[202]. In order for the world to move towards more clean power, countries, governments and businesses will have to make a switch to more renewable, sustainable and reliable sources of energy such as solar, wind, hydro, and/or biomass. Forward-looking governments around the world have been investing in renewable energy. Most governments are also strengthening investment conditions to spur private investment in clean energy. In this vein, governments are incentivizing investment in projects that use innovation to generate energy through renewable sources and reduce reliance on fossil fuels. These include the setting up of large-scale solar parks, wind farms, waste-to-energy plants, and big hydro-electric installations. According to the International Energy Agency's (IEA) Renewables 2017 report, renewable energy production surged in 2016, and two-thirds of net new capacity (amounting to approximately 165 gigawatts) is being generated through clean sources. China has been the growth leader in this area, and it is expected to account for more than 40% of the total global clean energy mix by 2022.[203] At the end of 2017, China deployed a number of innovative technologies such as a 100-meter tall tower that will suck smog and improve air quality in the city of Xian.[204] Similarly, in India renewable capacity is expected to more than double in the run up to 2022. In India, the growth in renewable energy has been driven by wind and solar, which represent 90% of India's capacity growth.[205]

In the Middle East, the United Arab Emirates has been playing a pioneering role in improving access to and generating clean energy from various renewable sources. The UAE government has spear-headed several ambitious initiatives in the renewable energy sector. The Shams Solar Park in Abu Dhabi is the Middle East's first utility-scale solar plant. Similarly, in Dubai, the Mohammed bin Rashid Al Maktoum Solar Park, which is currently in Phase 3, comprises of thousands of rows of solar photovoltaic panels. By 2020, this Park aims to generate

1000 megawatts of electricity, consequently powering 160,000 homes, and offsetting 1.4 million tons of carbon dioxide emissions.[206] Set for hand-over in 2025, Masdar City in Abu Dhabi aims to be the first zero-carbon city, with a capacity to house 50,000 people who will fully rely on renewable energy.[207]

While switching to a more renewable source of energy is a step in the right direction, it is not adequate for achieving sustainability goals. Energy needs to be delivered and stored in a way that minimizes wastage and cost without compromising on efficiency. Smart grids present a groundbreaking opportunity in this regard. They have an advantage over regular electricity transmission grids, in that they use digital technology to sense rapidly-changing demand for electricity. Decentralized smart grids that are connected to each other via cloud can enhance the efficiency, reliability, and asset utilization of an existing transmission grid[208]. Furthermore, the sensor-based technology of IoT, big data and analytics can be used to recognize and respond to demand without a lag. Demand and supply of renewables can be predicted using IoT and artificial intelligence. This has the potential to enhance energy storage and manage peak demand in a more streamlined manner[209].

Tesla Inc. (formerly Tesla Motors) is an example of a business leveraging 4IR technologies to produce and store renewable energy. Established in 2003 as a disruptive and innovative automaker specializing in environmentally friendly automobiles, Tesla aimed to vertically integrate across its supply chain. By 2012, Tesla had started exploring the opportunity to produce proprietary charging infrastructure as well as components [210]. Using its technological base from charging devices for electronic cars, in April 2015, the company unveiled its rechargeable lithium-ion battery stationary energy storage products for home and industrial use. The Powerwall was intended towards home energy consumers, who could use these batteries to store electricity for off-the-grid usage (for example, as back-up power or for load-shifting). On the other hand, Powerpack was a larger scale energy storage solution (storing 100 kWh of electrical energy) that could be used for integrating renewable power, peak load management, providing back-up power, and controlling voltage. In February 2017, Tesla signed a deal with Transgrid in New South Wales Australia to supply the state's homes with energy through Powerpacks. Another deal that Tesla signed in Australia was to build a 100 MW/129 MWh Powerpack system to provide an energy storage system for a wind farm near Jamestown, South Australia[211]. Not only is 4IR offering new technological solutions to our sustainability challenges, it is also opening up a new world of public-private partnerships in this domain.

In 2016, Tesla set up its first lithium-ion battery factory called the Tesla Gigafactory 1 in Nevada, USA, and in January 2017, the factory commenced mass production of cells. According to Tesla's CEO Elon Musk, a passionate environmentalist, the entire rationale behind the massive facility is to manufacture batteries that can be used to store renewable energy in a cost-efficient way[212]. Gigafactory 1's design is in itself a leading example of a state-of-the-art, eco-friendly production facility. To begin with, the facility is completely energy self-reliant. Powered by a 70-megawatt solar farm (with solar panels produced by SolarCity, which Tesla acquired in 2016), this all-electric facility will eventually have a rooftop installation which is seven times bigger than the world's largest rooftop solar installation. Furthermore, since no fossil fuels will be used to generate electricity, the facility will have no carbon emissions, and the building's heating will be provided by the waste heat emanating from the battery production process. The building will also feature a closed-loop water system that recirculates 400,000 gallons of water, thus using 80% less freshwater compared to standard processes. Tesla will also be able to recycle its battery cells into new cells on site via an onsite battery reprocessing facility[213].

Smart Transport

Transportation practices are one of the most important determinants of global sustainability. As global population, disposable income and urbanization increase, automobile dependence is likely to rise, thus exacerbating sustainability issues. Around the world, transport is a key challenge facing policymakers as they strive to achieve more sustainable development. This motorization crisis is particularly prevalent in urban contexts, where congestion and pollution levels are already high[214].

4IR technologies can be employed to create a paradigm shift towards more sustainable transportation models. Transport systems can be made smarter by harnessing the power of 4IR technologies such as 3D printing and advanced materials, which enable the production of lighter and more fuel-efficient vehicles. Moreover, these vehicles can be produced locally, further reducing the need for imports, transportation and ultimately, energy emissions. Advanced materials can also generate low/zero emissions automotive solutions, which can eventually replace vehicles that use combustion engines and rely on non-renewable energy sources. Autonomous drones and sensors connected to IoT platforms can create greater scope for optimized routing, as they enable real-time reporting of traffic and logistics information – ultimately leading to more sustainable transportation systems[215].

The recent breakthrough in autonomous vehicles has the potential to create innovative disruption in personal transport. By providing mobility-on-demand and vehicle sharing services, they can drastically improve the energy efficiency of road transport. Utilizing cloud and big data, these autonomous vehicles can communicate with transport infrastructure to facilitate better vehicle flows, eco-driving and road network efficiency. This innovation can have a large impact in industrial applications, as autonomous heavy vehicles (e.g. trucks and lorries) are safer, faster, and more energy friendly. As sensors and codes become more sophisticated, the technological obstacles (such as situational awareness of a vehicle versus a human driver) facing autonomous heavy vehicles will be overcome[216].

Founded in 2016, Otto is an example of an American company that is an industry leader ahead in implementing autonomous solutions for large vehicles. Otto outfits trucks with equipment that enables the trucks to drive themselves. The company is installing sensor and processing arrays on Volvo semis. The equipment installed comprises of four forward-facing video cameras, radar, and a cluster of accelerometers.

Most importantly, Otto installs a lidar system which uses a pulsed laser to collect detailed data about the truck's surroundings. The truck's inside is fitted with a micro super-computer that crunches extensive sensor data and adjusts the braking and steering commands according to the weight of the truck load. To turn the computer's output into actual commands for the truck, a drive-by-wire box has been installed. This box uses electromechanical actuators fixed to the truck's steering, throttling and braking systems[217].

Moreover, advanced materials technology can support the development of innovative solutions such as Hyperloop. Hyperloop is a high-speed vacuum-based mode of passenger and freight transportation. Designed jointly by Tesla and SpaceX (an American aerospace and manufacturer and space transport services company) to shorten the travel time between San Francisco and Los Angeles, Hyperloop is envisioned to be a transit system that consists of two reduced pressure tubes extending between the two cities. Capsule-shaped pods carrying passengers would travel through these tubes free of air resistance or friction conveying people or freight at super high speeds (circa 700 mph)[218]. The Hyperloop tubes will be powered through solar panels installed on the roof, thus being environmentally sustainable. Already out of the design phase and into piloting. Dubai, in the United Arab Emirates, will soon be home to one of the world's first Hyperloop pilot tracks.

According to estimates presented by the US Department of Transportation, Hyperloop routes can potentially be up to six times more energy efficient than air travel on short routes, and over three times faster than the world's fastest high-speed rail system. Another feasibility study conducted for the development of Hyperloop in Germany revealed that it would replace thousands of trucks from the road, thus reducing air and noise pollution, greenhouse gas emissions, traffic congestion and road accidents. While it may not be completely solar-powered, it still has the potential to avoid emitting up to 140,000 tons of carbon dioxide and up to 0.2% of Germany's entire production of air pollutants per annum[219].

Smart Cities

It is estimated that by 2050, 70% of the world's population will live in cities. In this context, sustainable urbanization and planning has to be prioritized by all governments around the world. While converting existing cities into smart cities is a complex task, 4IR technologies can facilitate this transition, and world cities today have many encouraging examples. Buildings and cities can leverage a range of 4IR technologies to enhance efficiency and generate environment-friendly outcomes. Each technology can contribute in its own way to reduce emissions and make construction and planning more innovative and green.

Cloud and big data, backed by IoT, are central for developing smart building systems that integrate heating, lighting and hot water. Cloud computing systems and sensors can be installed for quick and responsive home heating. They also offer cloud-based appliance control and digital planning processes. Furthermore, artificial intelligence can automate diagnosis and control systems and allow cue-responsive and remote management of water, lighting, appliance and heating usage. In addition. At the city level, IoT can also enable the development of efficient and eco-friendly energy use, water management and waste collection systems.

Advanced materials have the potential to improve the efficiency of the buildings. Efficient concrete, super insulation, and heat reduction are all areas within advanced material technologies offer the opportunity to customize building design to save energy and reduce the carbon footprint [220]. Construction can also be made more sustainable by employing next generation building codes that utilize digital design and nano-materials. This makes the construction process more efficient while also reducing carbon emissions in production[221].

Most importantly, 3D printing technologies are revolutionizing local building construction, particularly in the area of clean energy generation. These printing technologies also make solar energy more cost-efficient, as 3D-printed solar sprays enable the printing of solar cells on glass and other material surfaces, which enables them to generate their own energy[222].

On a more macro level, urban development planners can strategize and optimize city planning efforts to realize efficiency gains. Big data, open-source mapping platforms, augmented and virtual reality can be critical 4IR technologies in this regard. Sensors, smart meters and energy management systems can generate real-time data that can be used to optimize city-wide energy management (for example, managing peak demand for electricity, smart street lighting using renewable energy sources) as well as traffic management. These technologies offer great potential for making cities more responsive to the needs of the population, while being more sustainability-oriented[223].

The Danish capital city of Copenhagen is one of the pioneer cities that started collecting and employing big data and IoT to create a greener city. Backed by a detailed Smart City Plan, the Copenhagen city government uses data intelligently to address a range of urban development challenges. To manage traffic, parking sensors have been installed and taxi drivers (for example) pre-book parking spaces using smart phones. Moreover, waste collection has been optimized by using smart bins that monitor garbage levels in each bin and send optimized routes directly to municipality drivers when a bin is almost full. Air pollution monitors have also been installed in various parts of the city and data harvested through these devices is accessible to citizens through a mobile app. In the Copenhagen context, this is a critical development as 50% of workers and students cycle to work and the number of pedestrians is also high[224].

Environmentally conscious cities are also encouraging green innovation in building design and construction. The Singapore Government, for example, offers generous incentive schemes for innovative and digitized architectural design and energy-efficient technologies such as energy efficiency retrofits[225]. Furthermore, the Singapore Building and Construction Authority launched a building-rating and certification tool in 2005 to encourage investment in eco-friendly technologies such as computer modelling of energy flows and carbon emissions, water-efficient fittings, and motion sensors[226].

Sustainability is about balance

4IR technologies hold a lot of promise with regard to enhancing environmental sustainability, but there are some potential risks and unintended consequences associated with these technologies. In order to reap the maximum environmental benefits from the fourth industrial revolution, these risks have to be mitigated by the government, the private sector, and the citizens. For example, autonomous vehicles and vehicle sharing models (such as Uber) can trigger a rebound effect through reduced traffic and congestion. Car use can increase as private cars experience reduced journey times. Moreover, as the cost of autonomous vehicles declines in the face of increased competition, mass transit options may seem less appealing, thus leading to an increase in carbon emissions. This challenge can potentially be addressed by taking a policy stance to ensure that autonomous vehicles are low or zero-emissions. In addition, the rapidly growing digital economy that is driven by 4IR technologies can also generate additional greenhouse gas emissions and digital waste[227].

4IR technologies can also have negative social impacts such as loss of employment and challenges pertaining to data privacy and cyber security. The 2018 data issues with Facebook are a prime example. Governments and companies must ensure that these challenges are addressed to prevent citizen and consumer backlash. Government foresight and action are also required to re-skill the existing workforce and align education to meet future labor market demands. Thus, a responsive and agile governance structure has to be created to ensure that the fourth industrial revolution is sustainable and responsible[228].

4IR and the Future of Net Positive

Technology is redesigning the future of the world. Supported by data, 4IR technologies such artificial intelligence are ushering in a new era of connectivity and efficiency. This has far-reaching implications for business. The imminent change in the manufacturing process, and transportation and logistics will revolutionize the means and costs of production. However, businesses will also have to evaluate how their activities impact the social and environmental ecosystem. In order to ensure a steady supply of raw materials and improve revenue in a world of conscious global consumers and investors, businesses will have to align themselves with the sustainable development goals. Businesses will need to extend their sphere of influence beyond traditional corporate social responsibility models. Already consumers and investors expect businesses to monitor their economic, social and environmental impact, and take corrective action to control the damage they incur on a continuous basis.

In this scenario, businesses need to identify areas of maximum impact and design a targeted roadmap for delivering against the sustainable development goals. However, the alignment of business with the SDGs cannot come at the expense of the bottom line. In order to survive and generate profit, businesses will have to explore opportunity in areas that combine profitmaking with creating value for society and the environment. Companies are increasingly realizing the business case for engaging with the sustainable development goals, and moving beyond goals of merely reducing their carbon and water footprint. They are embracing the concept of being Net Positive, and creating business profits from solving social problems – an approach that is generating scalable and sustainable solutions to society's most pressing challenges. A Net Positive approach allows businesses to catalyze positive change across the value chain, and churn out a range of innovative products that give the businesses a competitive advantage and open avenues for profitmaking. In this scenario, the Sustainable Development Goals serve as a framework for Net Positive companies to make progress by providing a basis for materiality assessment, which helps identify areas that sustainability efforts should focus on.[229]

In this process of embracing a Net Positive approach, 4IR technologies have a critical role to play, and they must be leveraged to create long-term positive impact at minimum cost. These technologies will also help spur innovation in product development and allow businesses to effectively monitor impact as well as consumer sentiment. Businesses, both small and large, must learn from pioneering companies like Tesla,

General Electric and Philips, who have embraced the Net Positive approach not only to appear more responsible, but to truly integrate the concept into their business model. While new champions of Net Positive will face significant challenges with regard to quantifying and measuring impact, the cumulative value created by these businesses can nevertheless accelerate the achievement of the SDGs considerably.

(Endnotes)

175 The Fourth Industrial Revolution: What It Means and How to Respond. Klaus Schwab. Foreign Affairs. December 2015
176 Understanding the Internet of Things (IoT). GSM Association. ht t ps://w w w.gsm a .c om /iot /wp- c ontent/upload s/2 014 /0 8/ cl iot wp 07 14 .pdf. 2014.
177 An Introduction to the Internet of Things. Lopez Research. https:// w w w.cisco.com/c /d am/en us/solutions/trends/iot/introduc- tion to IoT november.pdf. November 2013.
178 Ibid.
179 Ibid.
180 Industry 4.0: The Next Industrial Revolution. IoT UK. October 2017
181 The Top 9 Augmented Reality Companies in Healthcare. Medical Futurist. HYPERLINK http://medica/ http://medica lfuturist.com/top-9-augmented-rea lit y-companies-healthcare/.
182 Uber launches Uber Health, a B2B ride-hailing platform for healthcare. TechCrunch. https://techcrunch.com/2018/03/01/ uber-launches-uber-hea lth-a-b2b-ride-hailing-platform-for- healthcare/. Mar 2018.
183 How to bring the excitement of a holiday to the high-street? http:// HYPERLINK http://www.alphr.com/samsung/1004971/how-to-bring-the-excitemen www.alphr.com/samsung/1004971/how-to-bring-the-excitemen t-of-a-holiday-to-the-high-street. December 2016.
184 How is 3D printing being used? TechWorld. https://w w w.tech- world. com/picture-gallery/tech-innovation/5-top-uses-of-3d-pri nting-3666509/. November 2017
185 Nike Jumping into 3D Printed Shoes with Prodways. All3DP. https://all3dp.com/nike-3d-printed-shoes-prodways/. June 2017.
186 Ibid.
187 Advanced Analytics Enhances Business Intelligence. Ventana Research. https:// HYPERLINK http://www.viftech.com/wp-content/uploads/2015/05/ www.viftech.com/wp-content/uploads/2015/05/ Adv a nc e d-A na ly t ic s -E n h a nc e s -Bu si nes s -I ntell i genc e -Ro bust-new-technology-enab.pdf. 2014
188 Industry 4.0: The Next Industrial Revolution. IoT UK. October 2017.

189 How Companies Learn Your Secrets. New York Times. https:// HYPERLINK http://www.nytimes.com/2012/02/19/magazine/shopping-habits.html www.nytimes.com/2012/02/19/magazine/shopping-habits.html. February 2012.

190 Ford Drives In The Right Direction With Big Data. Datafloq. https://datafloq.com/read/ford-drives-direction-big-data/4 34. July 2014.

191 The Amazing Ways Tesla Is Using Artificial Intelligence And Big Data. Forbes. ht t ps:// w w w.forb e s .c om/site s/ b er na rd- marr/2018/01/08/the-amazin g-ways-tesla-is-using-artificial-in- telligence-and-big-data/#ec46fa842704. January 2018

192 3 Advances Changing the Future of Artificial Intelligence in Manufacturing. Autodesk. https://w ww.autodesk.com/redshift/ future-of-artificial-intelligence/. January 2018.

193 Explaining AI: AI vs. Predictive Analytics. Magnetic. https:// HYPERLINK http://www/ www. magnetic.com/blog/explaining-ai-ai-vs-predictive-analy tics/. September 2017

194 Artificial Intelligence and Decarbonization. Anthropocene Magazine. HYPERLINK http://www.anthropocenemagazine.org/AI/ http://www.anthropocenemagazine.org/AI/. July 2017.

195 Smar t sensors w i l l detect env ironmenta l pol lution at t he speed of light. IBM. ht t ps://w w w.resea rch.ibm.com/5-in-5/ environmental-pollutants/.

196 DHL Trend Research & Cisco Consulting Services. Internet of Things in Logistics. 2015.

197 The Future of Jobs Employment, Skills and Workforce Strategy for the Fourth Industrial Revolution. World Economic Forum. http:// www3.weforum.org/docs/WEF Future of Jobs.pdf. January 2016

198 Dig it a l Div idend s – World De velopment Re p or t 2 016 . World Ba n k . HYPERLINK http://documents.worldbank.org/curated/ ht t p://doc u ment s .worldba n k .org /c u r ated / en /8969714 68194972881/pd f /102725 -PU B -Replacement- PUBLIC.pdf

199 Harnessing automation for a future that works. McKinsey & Company. January 2017.

200 Innovations for the Earth: Harnessing technological break- throughs for people and the planet. PriceWaterhouse Coopers. 2017

201 Ibid.

202 Renewable energy is not enough: it needs to be sustainable. World Economic Forum. https://w w w.weforum.org/agenda/2015/09/ renewable-energy-is-no t-enough-it-needs-to-be-sustainable/. 2015

203 Renewables 2017. International Energy Agency. 2017.

204 Three countries are leading the renewable energy revolution. World Economic Forum. https://w w w.weforum.org/agenda/2018/02/ countrie s-behind-global-renewable-energ y-grow th/. February 2018.

205 Ibid.

206 Why the UAE is betting big on renewable energy. Smithsonian Magzaine. https://www.smithsonianmag.com/sponsored/uae-betting-big-renewable-energy-180967320/. January 2018.

207 The UAE: A Pioneer in Renewable Energy. ADNOC. https://medium.com/@ADNOCdist/the-uae-a-pioneer-in-renewable-energy-94ada336b261. May 2017.

208 The Future of Electricity: New Technologies Transforming the Grid Edge. World Economic Forum. March 2017

209 Innovations for the Earth: Harnessing technological break- throughs for people and the planet. PriceWaterhouse Coopers. 2017

210 Tesla is now ~80% vertically integrated, says Goldman Sachs after a Tesla Factory visit. Electrek. https://electrek.co/2016/02/26/tesla-vertically-integrated/. February 2016

211 Tesla Just Landed a Deal to Build the World's Most Powerful Battery. Futurism. https://futurism.com/tesla-just-landed-a-deal-to-build-the-worlds-most-powerful-battery/

212 How Tesla And Elon Musk's 'Gigafactories' Could Save The World. Forbes. https://www.forbes.com/sites/ericmack/2016/10/30/how-tesla-and-elon-musk-could-save-the-world-with-gigafactories/#6079c30b2de8. October 2016

213 Tesla will power its Gigafactory with a 70-megawatt solar farm. The Verge. https://www.theverge.com/2017/1/11/14231952/tesla-gigafactory-solar-rooftop-70-megawatt. January 2017.

214 The Transport Challenge In The Sustainability Of Megacities. A. Igwe. Urban Transport XII: Urban Transport and the Environment in the 21st Century. Vol 89. 2006.

215 Innovations for the Earth: Harnessing technological break- throughs for people and the planet. PriceWaterhouse Coopers. 2017

216 Ibid

217 Self-Driving Trucks. MIT Technology Review. https://www.technologyreview.com/s/603493/10-breakthrough-technologies-2017-self-driving-trucks/. 2017.

218 Beyond the hype of Hyperloop: An analysis of Elon Musk's proposed transit system. New Atlas. https://newatlas.com/hyperloop-musk-analysis/28672/. 2013

219 'Faster, cheaper, cleaner': experts disagree about Elon Musk's Hyperloop claims. The Guardian. https:// HYPERLINK http://www.theguardian.com/ www.theguardian.com/sustainable-business/2017/aug/04/hyperloop-planet-environment-elon-musk-sustainable-transport. August 2017.

220 Innovations for the Earth: Harnessing technological break-throughs for people and the planet. PriceWaterhouse Coopers. 2017
221 Harnessing the Fourth Industrial Revolution for Sustainable Emerging Cities. World Economic Forum. November 2017.
222 3D Printed Solar Panels: The Next Step in the Renewable Energy Revolution. Greener Ideal. https://greeneridea l.com/ news/3d-printed-solar-panels/. April 5, 2016
223 Transforming cities for the better through sustainable technol- ogy. Siemens AG. 2013.
224 Copenhagen: The Great Dane of Sustainability. The Smart Citizen. https://thesmartcitizen.org/technology-enablement/copenhagen-the-great-dane-of-sustainability/. 2016
225 Sustainable Built Environment. Building and Construction Authority (BCA). https:// HYPERLINK http://www.bca.gov.sg/Sustain/sustain.html www.bca.gov.sg/Sustain/sustain.html.
226 Singapore Takes the Lead In Green Building in Asi a . Yale Environment 3 6 0. https : //e360.yale. edu/features /singapore takes the lead in green building in asia. 2013.
227 Innovations for the Earth: Harnessing technological break-throughs for people and the planet. PriceWaterhouse Coopers. 2017
228 Ibid.
229 Make it your business: Engaging with the Sustainable Development Goals. PwC. 2015.